How Concerned Should I Be?

Anandhi Narasimhan, MD
Child, Adolescent, and Adult Psychiatrist

How Concerned Should I Be?

Questions Pertaining to the Developing Mind

Anandhi Narasimhan, MD
Child, Adolescent, and Adult Psychiatrist

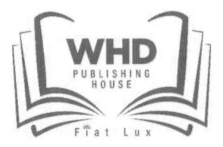

WHD Publishing House

Published by:
WHD Publishing House
#12/13, Karpagam Avenue,
4th Street, RA Puram,
Chennai – 600 028
www.whdph.com
Sales Headquarters – Chennai

Copyright © ANANDHI NARASIMHAN 2021

This book has been published with all reasonable efforts taken to make the material error-free after the consent of the respective authors. No part of this book shall be used, reproduced in any manner whatsoever without written permission from the editors, except in the case of brief quotations embodied In critical articles and reviews. The authors of the respective chapters of this book is solely responsible and liable for its content.

All rights reserved.

No part of this publication may be reproduced, transmitted or stored in any digital or electronic form. Also photocopying, recording or otherwise without the prior permission of the editor and publisher is strictly prohibited.

ISBN : "978-81-950109-4-3"
First Edition 2021
No. of Pages – 198

$ 22.99 USD

"Dr. Anandhi answers the questions caregivers have and tackles the important areas of development from childhood through adulthood. She is open, informative and honest. This book will feel like a conversation with a deeply knowledgeable friend!"

Marissa Leslie, MD,
Psychiatrist and Physician Executive

···•••••••···

"Dr. Narasimhan comes from a scientific background which helps her corroborate her clinical experience with the ability to critically appraise existing research, providing invaluable expertise with respect to issues affecting growing children, teenagers, and young adults. *How Concerned Should I Be?* translates that accumulated knowledge into language that is easy to understand and apply."

Sourish Saha, PhD
Senior Statistician

···•••••••···

"Dr. Anandhi Narasimhan's book makes her insight and expertise as an experienced child psychiatrist available at your fingertips. Her to commonly asked questions address a variety of issues throughout childhood, adolescence, and young adulthood. I highly recommend her book."

Rohan Calnaido, MD
Psychiatrist and Sleep Medicine Specialist

···•••••••···

"Based on my experience of counseling numerous expecting and new mothers when I was practicing as an obstetrician, I know that they needed a great variety of advice and guidance. I am happy to see Dr. Narasimhan's book How Concerned Should I Be?, which would have been valuable for those mothers and their families. This book is written in an easy-to-read, question-and-answer format; provides helpful advice to those who are raising their children from infancy through adolescence; and offers the nuanced perspectives necessary to address the needs of each child as an individual. The book should not only be helpful to parents, family members and guardians, but may also offer insight into the reader's own upbringing and reactions. I highly recommend it."

Manorama S Gupta, M.D.
Obstetrician and Gynecologist
President and Founder of Global Peace Foundation
Author of Mother To Be

•••••••••••••••

"Dr. Anandhi is an expert child psychiatrist, and I have had the opportunity to observe her empathic work with children, parents and treatment team members. She has written a book that is encouraging and thought provoking. It will open you heart and your mind as well as increase your knowledge. I would highly recommend it to parents and child caregivers."

Lorne Leach, LMFT, CADC-II
Program Director, Behavioral Health Services, Inc.

•••••••••••••••

"Dr. Anandhi is a very compassionate psychiatrist who takes the time to get to know her patients. She treats the whole person, and not just the symptoms and has a holistic approach to her psychiatric practice. In my role as a therapist, I was fortunate to consult with her about numerous dynamics that affected the families we treat. This book is so needed as it discusses issues that families experience as they navigate the development of their child through adulthood. This is a book I would recommend to everyone who is interested in learning more about how to approach future generations."

Yvans Jourdain, LMFT, Actor
Parks and Recreation, Grey's Anatomy, Judging Amy, The West Wing, Alias, Will & Grace

••••••••••••••••

"Dr. Narasimhan's book is a gift to both new and veteran parents. While it is not a substitute for professional advice, her insight from her own years of clinical practice to questions that many parents face is useful to help a parent get a dose of objectivity of their situation to help them pause, take a breath, and then proceed as more educated consumers of medical advice.

Her inquiry-based approach gives parents tools to probe to find root causes. I am impressed with the scope of the book, including considering multiple cultural and family backgrounds. She considers difficult situations and always offers compassionate and warm advice. She seems to virtually reach out and hold the reader's hand by assuring them that they are not alone by also revealing her own stories."

Dilip Barman
Whole food plant-based nutrition instructor
Executive Producer of "Code Blue" about lifestyle medicine

••••••••••••••••

CONTENTS

Acknowledgments — xiii
Introduction — xvii

PART ONE
The Early Years
Birth to 5 Years — 3

PART TWO
Childhood
6 to 11 Years — 45

PART THREE
Adolescence
12 to 14 Years — 85

PART FOUR
Late Adolescence and Young Adults
15 to 21 Years — 129

Conclusion — 165
References — 169

To my father, **_Dr. Krishna Narasimhan_**,
a scientist who loved his family.

ACKNOWLEDGMENTS

This book has been a culmination of numerous conversations, reflections, and reviewing existing research. I would like to thank my mentor Michael DeBellis, a renowned child psychiatrist researcher who introduced me to the field of child psychiatry through neuroimaging research. I would also like to acknowledge my many family members who supported me throughout this process. My parents were instrumental in motivating me to pursue academic and professional goals, providing a foundation based on encouraging a humble commitment to lifelong learning. The children in my family continued to give me inspiration while writing this book. Nancy Rosenfeld and David Tabatsky graciously contributed to helping me formulate the concept behind this book and taught me how to speak directly to people through writing. To my colleagues and friends, you have stood by my side over the years and celebrated every success. Thank you to my friends at World Humanitarian Drive, including Abdul Basit Syed and Sara Wilson, for keeping me on task and for helping me share this book with the world. Deepika Nimmagadda and Dana Rapneth helped me create a vision for the title of this book and I am grateful to their contribution. I am also grateful to my husband, David, who encouraged me to keep reaching for my dreams. Finally, this book would not have come into fruition without my patients, who continue to challenge me to approach problems with a compassionate mind; it has been truly an honor to be present with you in this journey.

"Don't worry that children never listen to you; worry that they are always watching you."

--Robert Fulghum, *Author*

INTRODUCTION

As a child psychiatrist, I hear many questions from parents who are worried about their children and want guidance on how best to manage the challenges they face with parenting. There are numerous parenting books that describe techniques with respect to setting limits, dealing with problematic behaviors, etc. This book may be interpreted as a deviation from a conventional "parenting" book in that it is more nuanced, with the goal of engaging people in a broadening of perspective approach, as opposed to an instruction manual. Development is a complicated interplay of numerous factors, and those magical transformative moments children have with adults are often less about a prescription and more about building meaningful connections.

To elevate consciousness, I wanted to offer transparency into some of the insights I have gathered over years of talking to parents and other adults who interact with children regularly, as well as talking to children in my role as a child psychiatrist. Child-rearing often involves innovation in how we think and is more of a journey rather than a destination. There needs to be an understanding of how to foster growth and autonomy while protecting children from damaging environments.

A child can be a mirror of our deepest fears, insecurities, and self-doubt. A child can also teach us about the beautiful purity of innocence, love, how to feel joy instead of fear, and offer an opportunity for profound emotional growth. I hope that some of these questions and answers are the beginning of a dialogue between adults on how to address various aspects of child development. It is not meant to be a one-stop shop with easy solutions, but instead hopefully will encourage approaching challenges with inquiry, seeking to understand the unique individuality of a child, and learning how to walk alongside children on their journey while holding their hand as needed.

·················

PART ONE

THE EARLY YEARS
BIRTH TO 5 YEARS

1. Do children have emotions at birth?

Newborn and infant emotional experiences are most commonly related to interactions that occur with a caregiver, such as during feeding, comforting, and holding.[1][2][3][4] A healthy baby starts moving well during this time and may even respond directly with a kick or a push to voices, singing, or music. Science tells us that a baby's smile, which first occurs two to three weeks after birth, is a sign of neurological activity but it does not necessarily mean the baby is "happy."[5] A social smile, which begins to happen after about three months, is more of a response to external stimuli, particularly looking at faces.[6] An important milestone occurs when a baby responds to a parent, like in a conversation, but with cooing instead of language. The American Academy of Pediatrics (AAP) recommends that parents sing, talk, play music, and read to their baby during pregnancy. There is also a suggestion that these behaviors and oral activities can lead to calmer babies and help a baby be more easily soothed by developing a previous inherent connection to his or her parents. Experts agree on the theory that a baby's facial expressions correlate with the development of his or her emotional state. This occurs in the context of interpersonal interaction with the primary caregiver. The difference in the development of emotions in babies versus adults is that emotional development in a baby is directly associated with physical and cognitive development.[7] The ability to truly feel these emotions happens later. A baby who seems "angry" before the age of six months is usually responding to a physical sensation of unpleasantness, as opposed to expressing what we would label as anger. Within three to six months, a baby develops experiential memories and begins to form expectations and frustration. Separation anxiety begins to happen around six to eight months, when a baby develops an awareness of strangers as well as attachments to caregivers, causing distress on separation.[8][9][10]

2. Our two-year-old son wakes up multiple times at night. My partner and I must go to work in the morning. The sleep deprivation is exhausting us. How do we deal with this situation?

Sleep deprivation is a big, often minimized risk factor for mental illness. Especially for new mothers, it is assumed culturally that it is par for the course for a woman not to sleep much after delivering a child. This adds to the fact that many women do not sleep well towards the latter part of the pregnancy or sometimes throughout their pregnancy. Sleep deprivation should not be minimized or dismissed because it can exacerbate existing mental illness or cause mental illness, often resulting in irritability, impaired functioning, etc.

In some eastern cultures after delivering a baby, relatives are supposed to come and help the new mother, so she gets time to rest. The pandemic also makes it harder because it involves taking a risk to let others come into their homes to help with childcare. It has been important to limit the number of contacts as part of the recommended public health measures. The issue of sleep deprivation is an important one and should be addressed. If it means allocating some resources to have help at night or during the day, that can be beneficial. Many women feel guilty if they are not breastfeeding, but one way to address sleep deprivation is to limit breastfeeding or incorporate a combination of breast and formula feeding to allow for some sleep.

As the child ages, encouraging a child's physical activity during the day may help with sleep training at night. Having a partner rotate schedules so that both parents do not have continued disruptive sleep can also be helpful, a luxury that is sometimes not available to single parents. Sometimes this is hard if you are living in a small, confined space and a crying baby or child wakes up both parents. Unfortunately, the demands of the workplace and financial responsibilities can make it hard to take time off work when you have not slept well at night.

Scheduled naps may have to be incorporated that give some uninterrupted time to rejuvenate the body. Having one parent that goes to sleep earlier so they get more sleep on the front end of the night may be a useful way to divided parts of the night. This is a lot harder in single-parent homes and those where partners do not have a solid working relationship and equal division of labor. Occasionally talking to a child's pediatrician or a mental health professional, such as a child psychiatrist can be beneficial in dealing with sleep-related issues. Sometimes there is utility in having a sleep study done for chronic sleep-related issues. Attending to a child's nutrition, not giving a child lots of sugar, especially late at night or food/drinks with caffeine are also measures to be taken into consideration as they certainly can affect sleep.

3. My three-year-old son lines up his toys obsessively, and he has trouble engaging with other children. What does this mean?

When a parent comes to me with a question like this, I must get a complete developmental history of their child. I like to begin by gathering information about the pregnancy, whether there were any complications, if the baby was born premature or at term, and if there were any issues with feeding or weight gain. Any one or a combination of these factors can be influential. Then I ask about developmental milestones, such as language, motor milestones, and socialization behaviors.

I try to assess for evidence of "joint attention," which is the ability of one person, even another small child, to engage another individual to direct their gaze by pointing to something, whether it is an object or a person. Joint attention is important in language development and comprehension. Studies show that problems with the development of joint attention are associated with developmental disabilities, such as autism. Neuroimaging studies suggest that there are certain areas of the brain that activate during joint-attention related tasks and that issues in these brain areas can be associated with Autism.[11] Delays in speech and language development do not necessarily mean the infant has an Autism Spectrum Disorder. It is important to know if the child's hearing has been tested, as hearing problems are known to cause speech and language delays.

As a child psychiatrist, I look for certain social skills during infancy, such as how an infant lets the caregiver know what he or she wants, how the infant interacts with others, and how the infant tolerates separation from the caregiver. Lining up toys is not necessarily always a sign of a problem, and the term obsessive is relative. When this type of behavior is combined with difficulty interacting with others or interrupts the child's functioning in other ways such as making transitions extremely hard, it warrants an evaluation by a

4. How do I help my child focus better and stay on task?

This is a great question especially in an era where there are so many distractions particularly digitally. The general recommendations regarding digital technology by the American Academy of Pediatrics are that a child should not have exposure to screen time for the first six months. Between six months to two years, it should be limited to social interaction with known adults and family members. Over the age of two until six it can be for educational content. It is important to know which type of educational content is useful because many of them may just be providing more unnecessary stimulation without a true education.

Digital platforms that encourage problem-solving and critical thinking can be used for educational content. Given the pandemic, children are spending more time on screens than ever. According to a report by Common Sense Media, prior to the pandemic, teenagers in the U.S. were spending on average of seven hours a day in front of screens which does not include time doing schoolwork. This is quite concerning because research shows us that time in front of the screen can affect posture, bone growth, contribute to the development of obesity which can lead to other metabolic problems.[12] Therefore, it is evident that the use of technology which has come with both benefits in harms must be balanced.

The digital platform is an area where predators use to seek out children to groom and victimize. It can also be a platform for cyberbullying, so it must be monitored and supervised. One challenge that parents have is limiting the amount of time in front of the screen. This may be difficult if children are doing most of their schoolwork on a digital device as has been happening during the COVID-19 pandemic. There are parental controls that can be used to limit

(text continues: "trained child mental health professional, such as a child psychiatrist or developmental pediatrician." appears at the top before section 4)

access to certain inappropriate content and to monitor how much time a child is using the device for things other than schoolwork.

A friend of mine told me if she found out her son was on his digital tablet for several hours during classes with virtual schooling. She was able to remove the device, so he did not have access, but it took a while to understand that was happening. When children grew up without cellular phones they played and engaged with other children without the use of a digital device. The availability of these technologies has also increased the anxiety of parents when they are unable to reach their child if the cellular phone battery dies or for other reasons.

Parents understandably want to know where their children are and be able to access them whenever needed. Although part of appropriate parenting involves parents knowing where the children are, who they are with, and what they are doing, there needs to be a balance where the phone is thought of as something extra for safety and to reduce the parent's anxiety, not increase it. In addition, many parents do not realize that even if they have a tracking device on their phone of their child, the child can leave the phone at a friend's house and still go places without the parents knowing. This gives the parents a false sense of security that the child is at home with a friend.

Even without the distraction of technology, about 7% of children have a mental health issue like Attention Deficit Hyperactivity Disorder (ADHD).[13] Many children can suffer from having trouble focusing, having problems staying still, being impulsive. For many of these children, early identification and intervention can really help. As humans, it is not biologically normal for us to sit in a classroom or front of a device for hours every day. There is a difference between having a normal restlessness when there are expectations of sedentary activity for prolonged periods, and hyperactivity that is associated with conditions like ADHD. For a percentage of the population, there are biochemical and morphological differences in the brain that make focusing and sitting still even harder in comparison to peers.

There are behavioral interventions such as providing frequent breaks, shorter assignments, more time to finish assignments as well as tests, and more individual attention which can make a huge difference.

When those interventions do not work, seeking the advice of a child psychiatrist or pediatrician that has received training in the treatment of ADHD can be beneficial. There is also some evidence that micronutrient deficiencies contribute to attentional problems sometimes the administration of certain integrative treatments can help. Sleep deprivation can cause problems focusing, and children with ADHD may also have an inherently harder time sleeping at night.[14]

The bottom line is even if your child struggles with a diagnosable ADHD disorder there are options to help them. It is also important that parents manage unrealistic expectations and appreciate the child's strengths. Sometimes those with hyperactivity symptoms find that an occupation that is more physically demanding works better for them. Michael Phelps the Olympic gold medal swimmer had a diagnosis of ADHD and his mother encouraged him to swim to address his hyperactivity. Gold medal gymnast Simone Biles also struggled with hyperactivity and inattentive symptoms. Getting physical exercise, eating a balanced healthy diet with focus on optimizing plant-based nutrition can help improve focus and concentration.

5. I am a new single mother, and I do not receive any child support. I feel utterly alone and scared about how I can manage this with two young children. How am I to manage being a good mom?

Being a single parent can be such a challenge. It is of great benefit to have at least one other person to lean on and share responsibilities of child-rearing. The other piece that is difficult for so many single parents is ensuring financial stability. Often single parents take on the entire financial burden of supporting a family which is a source of stress. However, having two parents that are unable to provide the proper care and nurturing of a child may be a worse situation than one parent who provides stability. There are some families where both parents are battling addictions or there is abuse which creates an adverse environment for a child. There are also families where the parents have multiple children without being able to care for them. Children can thrive in single parent homes if they receive the appropriate support. In many families, there is the tragedy where one (or both) parents pass away and the surviving partner or other caregiver is solely responsible.

The concept of single parents by choice is becoming more popular among women and men. There are different reasons for this. Some feel they have a dwindling biological clock and if they have not found a partner that they would want to have a child with they consider using a sperm or egg donor in the absence of a heterosexual union. For the LGBTQ population, using donor eggs, donor sperm, and the use of a surrogate allows them the opportunity to become parents. We are seeing a burgeoning of different kinds of families. There are concerns that arise around this; issues such as the use of the same donor for multiple offspring, potential psychological issues for donor-conceived people finding out later in life and feeling resentment as well as anger towards their social and biological parents.

The positive is that it may not be so taboo anymore to be a single parent in many circles although for women there still is quite a bit of workplace discrimination and sexism. There is still an ongoing misconception that a woman cannot balance both the career and children. In the book, *Marry Him*, author Lori Gottlieb makes a case for settling, the letting go of romantic fantasies. However, sometimes when we refrain from trusting our intuition, we can end up in situations that are not healthy for having a child and raising a child. In the same vein, we do not always know how things are going to turn out in the future so even well-intentioned efforts at avoiding risk may not be predictive of future success in relationships.

So many women and men may end up in abusive situations

which only causes adverse childhood experiences for their children. Many women and men have told me they did not see the abuse coming because early in the relationship as it was not visible, but the process of having children or other stress seemed to trigger the behavior. A person who has been victimized is more likely to be re-victimized, and many who grew up in abusive homes have found themselves in abusive relationships as adults. In these circumstances where abuse exists, separating and being a single parent may be the best thing for a child if abusive behavior cannot be curtailed. Also, there are other issues such as adultery, or a partner dealing with addiction, that can cause the fracture and dissolution of a relationship.

It can be useful to connect with a mental health or other non-profit agency that offers case management services. Having adequate childcare is often an issue among single parents. Joining support groups for single parents can provide a sense of community, facilitate trading of ideas and practical solutions for childcare, housekeeping, and offer emotional support. If one is sharing custody of their child or children, it can allow for some breathing room for self-care when the children are with the other parent. For those who do not trust the other parent, it becomes an additional source of stress when the children are away. Custody battles can become acrimonious with parents trying to spite the other and they can be ongoing, with numerous court proceedings when an amicable agreement cannot be sorted out.

Single parents can do very well if they are in the vicinity of supportive family members who are available for assistance. Often single individuals have the additional burden of caring for aging parents or other family members. We need to foster a sense of community and togetherness for single people specifically because much of world's population is in fact, single. There needs to be understanding at the workplace that if a child is sick, there may not be another parent readily available to pick the child up from school or take care of that child for the day. A child may have special needs, mental or physical conditions that require frequent appointments that the single parent must be available for. Financially supporting the family is imperative, so having a job is vital and not optional for so many single parents. There are government programs in various parts of the world that are available to provide food and other resources. Spiritual houses of worship can also be a resource to single parents if they are supportive environments. A child raised with a single parent can still have a thriving, abundant childhood, develop meaningful committed relationships in the future, and have a bright outlook.

6. I have noticed that my daughter does not smile anymore, what could be causing this?

This is a scenario that prompts inquiry from me. Was the child smiling before? When did this start? Was there any sort of stress that precipitated this? Sometimes a precipitating stressful experience can affect a child's mood and social expressions. If there has been trauma a child may lose the ability to find enjoyment and it is expressed as a reduction in smiling. It is important to be aware of whether there is any abuse happening. Family stresses, medical illnesses in the family, natural disasters like fires and storms can precipitate feelings of stress in a child. Bullying can also be a source of stress and impede a child's ability to feel enjoyment.

Children, even at a young age, can experience depressive symptoms. This may include not smiling, crying frequently without cause, irritability, lack of interest in things, fatigue, trouble sleeping, and appetite disturbances. They may also have trouble with concentration and interacting well with others. It is also important to evaluate for any developmental issues. Children who have trouble with social cues or communication with others may have a developmental issue that is worth further evaluation by a developmental pediatrician or trained mental health professional familiar with developmental disorders. There is also genetic component of depressive disorders, it can run in families and a child may have a genetic predisposition to the development of mood disorders like depression. There are evidence-based therapies that can help with children who suffer from depression or trauma. Access to these resources is important.

7. I cannot seem to get my son to eat green vegetables. I know it is important for a child to have a healthy diet with lots of nutrients. How do I encourage my child to eat healthy food like vegetables?

Children should have a diet that incorporates healthy vegetables and fruits. Dark green vegetables have an abundance of nutrients that are helpful for both brain development and disease prevention.[15][16] I often get the complaint that a child does not want to eat healthy food. Forcing a child to try and eat the same thing repeatedly may make them averse to eating it in the future, so one way is gradually introducing the healthy option, presenting it to them over time as a choice. Another option is becoming creative like mixing spinach or kale and other nutritious vegetables and fruits in a smoothie, to camouflage the taste of certain things that a child does not like. Certain fruits such as mangos and watermelons have a high sugar content, so substituting them for others such as blueberries, blackberries, and raspberries can help moderate the amount of sugar a child receives.

For children who have difficulty with certain textures and even the color of certain food, this can continue to be challenging. The food battle is often an exhausting one for parents. There are certain shakes available that provide some of the nutrients your child may be missing (it is important to be aware of sugar content in these also).

Also understanding a parent's limitations is important. Parents also often pressure to be able to do it all, work, cook healthy meals, manage various tasks as a parent, especially for mothers who in many cultures still face inequality with the division of labor. Frozen vegetables may be a good substitute for fresh vegetables when parents feel they do not a lot of have time to prepare food. In many parts of the world, access to refrigeration makes it paramount that fresh vegetables and fruits are utilized soon. Every child should have access to healthy food worldwide. Adopting a more plant-based lifestyle rich in whole foods can help the future wellbeing of your child. There is research showing that micronutrient deficiencies can contribute to attention difficulties and mood and anxiety issues, so when this is addressed, it can help a child's mental health as well.

8. Can integrative medicine play a role in my child's health?

Integrative medicine can play a significant role in a child's health, in fact, it is imperative. There is a shift from what was previously called alternative medicine to integrative medicine because this aspect of medicine should not be mutually exclusive from allopathic treatments. The medical education system is often devoid of nutritional training which is an important factor when considering disease prevention and management. For example, we have learned over time that it is important to limit salt when there is high blood pressure. Balanced nutrition should play a role from the beginning not just after the presentation of an affliction.

The American diet has been infiltrated by processed foods, additives, and fast food. Blueberries, raspberries, blackberries have antioxidants that booster immunity. As already mentioned, there is research showing that micronutrient deficiencies can contribute to additional difficulties and mood and anxiety issues.[17]

Medical conditions like anemia or thyroid imbalances can also contribute to mental and physical health issues, so iron deficiencies or thyroid related hormonal abnormalities must be corrected. I have treated children who present with fatigue and depression, and when I order lab work, I find that they are anemic. Often, when we correct things like anemia the mental health symptoms may also improve. Deficiencies in micronutrients like magnesium can affect attention issues.[18] There is data that omega-3 vitamins (which come either from fish sources or plant-based sources like algae) can help with cognitive functioning such as attention and mood stabilization.[19]

Melatonin is a supplement that we already have in our bodies, a little extra can be an option for children who have trouble falling asleep.[20] Integrative treatments can be discussed with a professional who specializes in this type of intervention. Integrative treatment also involves incorporating daily physical activity for children to promote their growth and help them thrive physically and mentally.

9. My husband has an alcohol problem and does not think he does. I just want him to get some help. My son sees him under the influence. How will this affect him?

Substance abuse and dependence is a monumental problem worldwide. Millions of people struggle with this and as with a lot of things related to health, the issue of substance abuse is on a spectrum. Let us take the example of alcohol use as it pertains to this question. The same concepts I will be illustrating can be applied to other forms of drug use. Some individuals participate in occasional social drinking, there are those who engage in binge drinking, and there are those who feel the need to drink heavily daily. Given that alcohol is a legal substance, it is accessible and readily available. It is also considered socially acceptable at business dinners, at family and social gatherings, and while watching sporting events in many cultures. Drinking can sometimes help people who have social anxiety being more engaging.

There is an abundance of research showing the link between heavy alcohol use to numerous medical conditions such as heart disease, cancers, strokes, liver dysfunction, etc.[21] There is also a growing climate on college campuses with more binge drinking and alcohol toxicity. Working a demanding job, providing for a family, parenting, family dynamic issues, and responsibilities such as caretaking, are examples of stress that can take an emotional toll, so many people often turn to alcohol to cope. Sometimes people drink because they simply like the way it makes them feel, or they like that they can socialize with less anxiety in social situations. Others enjoy drinking alone and take solace in being able to escape reality. When alcohol use is excessive, it can affect one's functioning, it can negatively affect health, and cause problems in interpersonal interactions.

When I talk to children whose parents have dealt with alcohol abuse or dependence, I get a variety of responses. For some, their parent is "a happy drunk," is easy to get along with when drinking, and may just drink while watching TV without causing a lot of disruption. The spouse or partner of the one who is drinking may feel stress when they see how much is being consumed, but the child may be shielded if they do not see much of a change. This could also be because of the development of tolerance to the point that someone can drink a lot of alcohol without feeling the effects of intoxication, and people around them may not notice a difference in their disposition.

Alcohol abuse and dependence is something that requires reflective insight and the acknowledgment that it is a problem. A loved one may gently bring it up as an issue that needs to be addressed and sometimes effective communication can help to motivate the individual with the drinking issue to make changes or seek help. At other times, often to the frustration of the partner, the individual continues the drinking behavior and is not able to be fully present as a parent or a partner and they may even put family members at risk. For example, a parent that is drinking may be forgetful or not pay attention to the needs of the child they are responsible for when the other parent is away.

Far too often there are stories of adults becoming verbally aggressive or violent when drinking, causing psychological or physical harm to the other family members. Adverse childhood experiences that precipitate stress can damage a child's physical and mental health. Dealing with the instability of a parent with a drinking problem can also cause trauma for a child, especially if abuse happens. If the adult who has a drinking issue is in denial, the partner can seek support from organizations like Al-Anon, which provides support for family members affected by alcohol and drug use. Family members can communicate with those who have been in the same position and learn other ways to get help.

If there is abuse or neglect happening, or a child is put in danger such as when a parent who drives under the influence, sometimes an agency like child protective services needs to be involved to protect children, and a court-appointed judge may order the drinking parent to get treatment. Many nations do not have an organized system to adequately protect children, and even when there is a system, there can be huge gaps in effectiveness. Ultimatums such as threats of separation can sometimes work to get a partner with alcohol issues to seek help, but sometimes they do not. The chaos alcohol and drug abuse can bring to the family can be very disruptive and damaging. There is also an increase in suicide attempts when substance abuse is in the picture.[22] If the individual with the problem is not willing or agreeing to get help, and if they do not minimize use themselves, then the partner can find resources for themselves. Individual therapy, and support groups can be vital in helping to understand substance abuse and what to do about it.

10. My four-year-old has a lot of difficulty with transitions. For example, if he is engaged in one activity, like playing with his toys, he has a tantrum whenever I tell him it is time for bed. Why does this happen?

Having some difficulty with transitions is developmentally appropriate at young ages. As infants grow, they begin to sense frustration and often have tantrums as an expression of those feelings. Children with speech delays may get frustrated more easily because they struggle to communicate. When a child goes to daycare or school for the first time, he or she usually faces some type of developmentally appropriate difficulty with the transition. Most children experience at least a little initial trouble separating from their parents. Gradually, they become more comfortable with the transition. For many parents, putting their child to bed is challenging, especially when a child does not want to settle down for the night or is not able to easily. Adequate exercise and activity during the day help to expend physical energy so that a child feels sufficiently tired by the evening. Long naps during the day often make it difficult for a child to fall asleep at night. The amount of nap time versus uninterrupted nighttime sleep can vary with different children, so often it takes time to understand what schedule works the best. Children with attention-deficit hyperactivity disorder can have difficulties with sleep and transitions.

Those with autism can also have these challenges. If the tantrums and difficulty with transitions seem more than age-appropriate, it may be helpful to seek an evaluation by a child developmental pediatrician, child psychiatrist, or a professional who understands developmental issues. Autism is not only defined by difficulty with transitions; it is a feature of autism. Difficulty with transitions in the absence of other social difficulties, or rigidity alone, does not necessarily imply that the child has autism. A child expert who has training in identifying developmental delays and Autism Spectrum Disorders can help distinguish this for you. Difficulties with transitions can be triggered by stress as an expression of a child's anxiety. Transitions can be difficult when parents separate, children go back and forth between two homes, sleep in different beds, and adjust to alternate settings. If hostility and verbally aggressive behavior exist at home, and domestic violence occurs, a child may display great difficulty with transitions. Sometimes this challenge is time limited, and it gets better over time. One way of handling tantrums is to de-escalate a child by not yelling at them, instead giving the child some space. Remove things in the vicinity that he or she can throw and make sure that the child is not hurting themselves. If a child is engaging in head-banging or hitting their own body, a more urgent evaluation or speaking with the appropriate professional is warranted.

11. My husband recently found out he has a child with another woman. How do we share this information with our daughter?

Marriages often do not necessarily play out like the fairytales young people are sold about it. Marriages can be a great source of comfort, stability, security, and wellbeing when they are healthy and functional. This scenario can confront the marriage with a challenge, and many families have had to grapple with how to deal with this kind of life-altering information. For some fathers, they are notified about a child of theirs as the child ages, but not necessarily as a call to be involved in the other child's life. It may simply be the mother felt the obligation to let him know or to seek financial child support. It may also be very possible that the mother wants her child to have a father who is an active participant in parenting, and the father wants the same.

This news is often shocking for the father to find out. He may have lots of emotions, he may experience a lot of guilt for not being more responsible at a younger age, and he may grapple with worries about what to do next. This also may affect the family concerning finances involving supporting another family, emotions on the part of the woman finding out about her husband's other child, causing her to feel emotions like anger and disappointment. For the woman who finds out about this, it is often a shattering of her image of an intact family. There also can be societal implications on how to disclose this information to communities of family and friends or whether to keep it a secret, which can be difficult. It also means that children can find out they have siblings they did not know existed, which can be like the experience by donor-conceived children (although the emotional landscape of the family may be vastly different at the time of discovery).

The first step needs to involve a resolution or healing between the parents after finding out about the existence of another child. This may be a fluid process with respect to healing communication and resolution of hurt. It can be hard to keep emotions and conflict away from children, and children often hear their parents argue or hear their mother crying about painful emotions that she is feeling. Children often feel the need to protect their mother and may show expression of anger at the father. Sometimes this type of information coming out can fracture a family without repair which becomes a dynamic the child has to learn to navigate. Whatever is the eventual outcome, it is so important to keep the children's emotional growth and health in mind.

It is important to have open honest communication with your child that is in a developmentally age-appropriate dialogue. It is also important to offer them comfort and reassurance that their feelings are being validated as well. Children may feel confused because it also alters their perspective of what a family looks like, they may feel excited to find out they have another sibling, but also feel guilty about that excitement and need to conceal it because their parents may not be happy about it. I have seen situations where the mother who finds out about this is forgiving, accepts the situation, and is willing to assist her spouse in figuring it out. A woman may process her emotions, encourage her partner to take responsibility for his previous actions, and consider the needs of his other child. Sometimes it leads to feelings of not getting enough attention for her child which is a dynamic that can happen in blended families.

With good communication and a secure, trusting relationship between the partners, this circumstance can be worked out to the harmony of all involved. If there does not exist infidelity in the current relationship and a woman can accept that her husband had this happen as part of his past, she may feel like this is a situation that just needs to be addressed. A therapist can help navigate difficult communications between the partners and the children. When there is added mistrust or active infidelity, or even the existence of situations where other women claiming that her husband is the father of their children and it is found to be true, this may just be too hard to handle. It is important to also acknowledge that infidelity and multiple sexual partners increase the risk of the development of a variety of sexually transmitted diseases, especially if one does not use adequate sexual protection. It is not just with professional athletes or some politicians that this phenomenon happens. Worldwide some men have children with multiple women. In some cultures, this is culturally sanctioned and is the norm. Also, the norm in many cultures is that a woman does not have any freedom or rights to demand things be different, nor can she engage in such behaviors herself. She may be shamed for feeling uncomfortable, and often forced into a family setup she would not otherwise desire. This can all contribute to the disempowerment of a young woman, leaving her psychologically bereft and resigned to relationships she would not choose to have. Even despite all this, women may still seek their own empowerment by getting involved with different partners in reaction, taking potentially grave risks for freedom.

Whatever one's personal beliefs are concerning this type of non-nuclear family system, a woman can work on her empowerment and think about how to best address the needs of herself and her child. Children deserve to experience healthy family dynamics. That does not mean mollifying or diminishing your voice, and not being assertive (except in abusive relationships when speaking up or not speaking up both result in violence, this needs support and resources to help a woman escape). There can be room for growth, and honest, open exchange between people can result in efforts to work together for happiness. In the animal species, there is research showing that some male members of the species mate with females of different "tribes" to propagate a species from an evolution standpoint.[23,24,25] Men with chauvinistic attitudes like to use the biological imperative as a justification for their infidelity without taking personal responsibility for their actions. It can often make a woman feel humiliated or ashamed to hear this kind of language. The reality is also that women can be just as guilty of having different partners or infidelity in places in the world where women have more freedom. We do not have to look at men and women as two different football teams fighting against each other with conflicts of interest. Instead, we should look at unions as an opportunity for growth in intimacy and as a potential for real emotional and spiritual growth.

12. When we go out in public, my four-year-old son has panic attacks. How do I help him deal with his anxiety?

Anxiety is an emotion that serves a function in the normal fight or flight response to perceived threats of danger. From an evolutionary perspective, anxiety was helpful to help us be aware of imminent danger such as with predatory animals. With the advent of weapons and shelter, there has been more space between us and wildlife as well as some natural threats. Weather-related dangers, food and water scarcity, and lack of shelter are real-life concerns for migrants and others worldwide.

Anxiety can help protect us in these situations by keeping us vigilant for dangers. For example, if you fear getting burned you learn not to put your hand in the fire. Stranger anxiety can begin in an infant around six months of age.[26] This is a normal developmental process where the infant seeks comfort from a known parent or caregiver and will often cry when picked up by someone else. Separation anxiety also becomes apparent when children start going to school. They may cry when parents drop them off or they are put in a daycare or with the babysitter. Children may also express anxiety by crying or being fearful if there is mistreatment, so it is important to notice changes in behavior that may be due to this. Instead of something bad going on, by and large, some separation anxiety and social anxiety are developmentally appropriate.

However, if a child continues to have panic attacks which may include a racing heartbeat, sweating, a sense of impending doom or difficulty breathing, this may be indicative of an anxiety disorder. Children can also exhibit anxiety by complaining of stomachaches or headaches, having sleep disturbances. Anxiety can be treated with evidence-based therapeutic interventions and occasionally medication if needed if it greatly impacts the child's functioning. Teaching a child how to engage their breath in helping them to calm down, how to distract themselves, and increasing focus on grounding techniques can all help with the panic attacks. Often the panic attacks can be exacerbated during a time of stress. One example is if the child is involved or witnesses something like a car accident. They may have anxiety afterward, sleep disturbances, and worries about getting into an accident every time they are in a car. This may be an adjustment process that gets better over time. If this is an ongoing issue, therapeutic intervention can be helpful. Therapeutic techniques taught early on can also allow the child to have learned coping skills so they can better deal with anxiety and have a role in the prevention of the development of mental health illnesses like anxiety disorders.

13. Our five-year-old son has leukemia and is now in remission. I have not been as attentive to his older brother during his sibling's treatment, and he seems to resent me for this. How do I show him love, while I am also continuously worried about his brother's illness coming back?

Research on major medical illnesses in children shows that often the parents may develop anxiety, depression, posttraumatic stress disorder.[27] Siblings also can develop symptoms of anxiety, depression, and posttraumatic stress disorder.[28][29] Depending on their age and level of comprehension, they may not understand they may not understand how sick their sibling is, or the concept of impending death if the illness is terminal. They may be confused as to why when their sibling gets a cold, it may result in hospitalization and why they may not recover quickly. They also may not understand why their sibling needs protection even when they look healthy, and why the parents are so worried about keeping their sibling from getting sick. They may not understand why they cannot play with their sibling or why there is an added level of punitive action if they play a little rough with their sibling. It is also hard for the parents to resume life as normal in the face of chronic uncertainty about the well-being of the child.

Chronic illness does not allow for recovery like that which can occur with acute illness. As a result, there is often a constant level of anxiety, that parents feel which increases their stress and is felt by the other child. The sibling may also feel guilty that he or she is healthy and does not have the same affliction. They may even feel jealous and wish that they were the ones who are sick so that they could get the same level of attention. They may feel depressed or anxious which may be reflected in their school performance or their behavior with other children. It is not uncommon for children to express themselves by acting out, having sleep disturbances, appetite disturbances, stomachaches or headaches, and poor school performance. This may be because they are unable to express their emotions and know how to cope. In situations like this, the sibling must receive therapy to help them cope with the situation.

Even though having a sibling with chronic illness is a tragic experience for the family to go through, there can be some positivity for siblings. They often grow up to have lots of compassion for human suffering because they had to learn to adjust to it when they were young. They may join support groups and be of help to others who experience similar situations. Finding support groups for siblings of children with chronic illnesses can be helpful so that the other sibling does not feel alone. Reminding them that you care about them just as much and that you want them to feel loved is important.

It can be a value for a parent, to be honest with their child. You can say, "Yes, mommy is worried about your brother's health but that doesn't mean that I love you any less. I am sorry if I do not always seem cheerful or if I am unable to do all the things that we would want to do together as a family. You are being strong to have to deal with this as well and I know it is not easy. We will deal with it together as a family and we will work together to support each other because that is what families do."

Role modeling to the sibling of the child dealing with the medical illness is important because you also want both children to try to feel some sense of normalcy even with what they are going through. Being in remission from leukemia or other cancers may mean that children can be involved in playing games together as a family and doing fun things with their sibling. This allows them normal childhood moments of joy and an abundance of fun. Focusing on giving both children that kind of experience despite your anxiety can be of great value to both. As adults we want to constantly reflect on our coping mechanisms and ability to be there for children. Getting family members involved that you trust or good friends who can offer the sibling extra support and attention can help the sibling not feel neglected when you are not available due to doctor's visits and hospital stays. Having a sick child can also cause a lot of stress in a marriage, and sometimes disagreements on care, blaming of the other parent for not doing enough at the right time can fracture the relationship. Checking in with the other parent and turning towards each other for support can help build the bond during difficult times.

14. My five-year-old overheard our babysitter say that people are killing each other in her native Honduras. How do I talk to him about this?

It is important to try and shield young children from a lot of this information as it can be traumatic and foster fear as young children cannot process these themes well. Sometimes it is hard to shield your child completely from these conversations as in this case. It is good to discuss this with your nanny and explain to her that you would rather not have this kind of content be discussed with your five-year-old. You do not want to belabor this story with your child, nor do you want to be dishonest, but you can say "yes, sometimes bad things happen in the world but there are a lot of good people who are working together to keep the world safe." You do not want to expose your children to graphic content or imagery. As they get older, they learn about violence in schools and talking to other people, but they should not be flooded with this at a young age before they can know how to process it and compartmentalize it. Nowadays, there is also more graphic content that is easily consumed. A child can learn about things without having to see footage of violence that can be traumatizing. You do not want them growing up thinking that their world is a violent one and there is no escape from it. It removes their sense of control over their living experience.

15. My partner is hesitant about vaccinating our baby because he heard some propaganda about all vaccines being dangerous. I want my child vaccinated as I know it is important to prevent the development of diseases. How can we come to an agreement on this?

Over the past decade, I have heard this question more and more as the anti-vaccine movement has gained traction, especially online, on social media platforms, and on dubious websites run by people who seem keen on spreading around conspiracy theories of all kinds. Anti-vaxxers are people who view vaccines as a dangerous violation. In 2013, we saw a 12 percent increase in Texas in the US of parents refusing vaccines for their children, and according to a review by the National Institutes of Health, this led to the largest outbreak of pertussis (whooping cough) since 1959, with nearly 4,000 cases reported just in that year. This is just one example of how dangerous refusing vaccines can be. In 2000, the highly contagious measles virus, was thought to be eliminated, due to a certain vaccine program that was implemented. However, there has been a relatively recent resurgence of measles, which has created huge public health concerns. It is often dire for children who are immunocompromised to be around unvaccinated children, as they are much more susceptible to the development of such infections.

A child can be immunocompromised due to cancer, metabolic illness, immunological diseases, or because of medical treatments that tax the body and deplete the physical resources needed for a strong immune system, such as chemotherapy. What makes this especially dangerous is that many of these vulnerable kids look quite "normal" and can easily be infected by unsuspecting, unvaccinated children whose parents do not even know that their child is hosting a possibly lethal infection until it is too late.

Anti-vaxxers often believe that vaccines will cause Autism or other brain diseases. Despite the lack of evidence of this, we still see widespread propaganda influencing parents to refuse vaccinations. The American Academy of Pediatrics and the Centers for Disease Control (CDC) have been educating parents about vaccines and encouraging them to discuss their concerns with their child's pediatrician. The CDC estimates that over 21 million hospitalizations and 732,000 deaths have occurred over 20 years from people not adhering to well-established guidelines for administering vaccinations. Now with the coronavirus pandemic, there is similar propaganda being spread about COVID-19 vaccinations which is causing many people to fear getting the vaccine.

Simply telling your partner that he is wrong about his position on vaccines may not be effective, especially since the anti-vaccine propaganda movement is built on elevating fear around vaccination. Instead, research shows that a more effective approach towards changing anti-vaccine attitudes involves providing information about the dangers of communicable diseases.[30] Having a discussion with your partner and your child's pediatrician can allow the pediatrician the opportunity to explore your partner's concern and address misinformation.

16. Being a vegetarian, I want my children to grow up the same way, but my partner does not. How do I convince her it is healthier for our children?

Diet is often influenced by culture, religious beliefs, ethical values, and upbringing. There can be a real difference in value systems concerning eating meat. For many people being vegetarian or vegan also feels more spiritually aligned with the concept of compassion towards all living things. However, for those who eat meat, it may be important to them that they continue to have this as part of their life for different reasons. They may like the taste of meat, they may associate meat with cultural traditions around food and home cooking, they may feel it gives them more protein and helps them manage weight. They may also just not want to compromise on things they enjoy for the sake of a relationship. Many people do not go a day without eating meat.

One way to discuss this is to share some information with your partner. There is definitive research that meat is associated with a lot of different cancers.[31] [32] There is also the issue of hormonal influences on animals and the processing of meat which can have deleterious effects on our bodies.[33] It can be a source of stress when one parent wants their child to have a different diet compared to their partner. This is one of those things that should be discussed in detail and to see whether it is possible to join on some common ground. Maybe you eventually agree to occasionally allow your children to eat meat at restaurants. Maybe you both agree on not having it in the home. Maybe in the process of sharing educational materials, you teach your husband more about some possible benefits of incorporating a more plant-based diet. There are a lot of people who grow up in families that do eat meat and later they decide they do not want to eat meat.

Another avenue is to share your values with your children about why you do not want to eat meat and why you would hope that they adopt a more plant-based lifestyle. As children grow, they may refuse certain parts of the diet. Either they do not like the taste or as they grow up it seems to feel better to them ethically to avoid meat as they start to understand how animals are treated. Depending on geography and culture sometimes is easy or easier to be vegetarian. Explaining to your husband why this is important to you may make him want to accommodate some of your values. This issue may also be symbolic of how flexible and compromising your partner can be even before marriage. If they can try to understand things from your point of view, validate you, and work to try to make sure you feel your values are respected, that is ultimately great for the marriage.

17. My husband's siblings do not visit or keep in touch with us much at all. It hurts me that my children do not have a close relationship with their aunts and uncles or their cousins. How can I talk to them about this?

The blending of families can be stressful in a marriage and there can be a lot of strife. Also, there may be different ideas of what different individuals want in terms of spending time together. Sometimes it is a logistical issue such as the geographical distance that gets in the way. Other times people feel like they have a lot on their plate, and they do not have much energy or interest in spending that much time with other family members. It may also be that the spouse does not feel comfortable with their partner's family members so that could also be a reason that they keep a distance. Sometimes it is not personal at all, people can get busy and time flies by.

There are dynamics in family systems where some individuals crave more time and attention and others do not. Unfortunately, it can affect children. Children may enjoy hanging out with their cousins but because the parents do not get along, they do not get to do so as much as they would like. Sometimes people feel like they are being asked to babysit without appreciation or gratitude. Single people and couples without children may not want to engage that much if they do not have children of their children. Sometimes people are not even aware that you feel like this, and it may be a matter of a simple conversation. You can say "I love it when you spend time with my children, and I would love for them to have a close relationship with you. Is it possible that we can work out a schedule that is comfortable for you where are you get to spend quality time with them?"

If you do not feel like you are getting much from the other party, it may be useful to then focus on other sources of socialization for your children. The COVID-19 pandemic has made it hard for extended families to connect and spend a lot of quality time together. That has become an additional challenge for fostering connection. This does involve some creativity and innovative thinking; whether it is having family virtual meetings or socially distanced meetings outdoors, so that the children can interact with family members and family members living alone do not feel isolated.

18. I am Catholic, and my husband is Jewish. We disagree on how to raise our children with respect to faith. He does not want baptism and I do not want my children to spend a lot of time in Hebrew school distracted from other things. How can we best raise children in an inter-religious home?

Religious differences can be a source of discord, but it does not have to be. We live in a world where there is a diversity of faith, and those of different faiths should be able to live harmoniously together. How religion is practiced can be individualized and different people participate in faith-based activities at different degrees. Where it becomes a conflict in relationships happens when there is disagreement in how much time is spent participating in religious activities and which religious faith to practice and how much.

For some couples, there is a mutual understanding that their children are exposed to both faiths, and how that is done is agreed on. This tends to work well when neither partner is super fixated on ritualistic elements. If there is mutual understanding between partners on the level of exposure it can work well. It is also important that the religious community is welcoming of the other partner so that they feel they are part of an inclusive environment. This is not always possible. Have a conversation with your wife about how you feel and what aspects are important to you concerning religious faith. In couples of different faiths, you can come to an understanding of mutual respect and a shared resolution of how to introduce different faiths to children.

Religion and racial differences can often create some tension with respect to parenting. I do believe that interracial and interreligious unions are an important part of societal progression. How else do we heal pain besides through loving one another through differences? Although having commonalities around race and religion can sometimes make it easier for people to be on the same page concerning what they want to expose their children to, sometimes only focusing on that may cause you to overlook some other problematic behaviors. Also, there is an issue of the degree that people want their children to be involved in religious activities. For some religions such as Hinduism or Buddhism, the spiritual focus on self-realization requires self-reflection and meditation which does not necessarily require being collectively involved in a community to practice the religion. Other religions or aspects of religions may be more bit insular and exclusive of other faiths and their practices. These are useful discussions to have ideally before having children but even during the process of raising children.

There are benefits to being involved with a house of worship such as the sense of community, sense of belonging, a place to focus on spiritual and personal growth, and a venue where children can be taught some of the values that their parents believe in. It is possible to expose your child to different religions and if done correctly, they can potentially grow up to appreciate the beauty of different faiths, leading them to respect people for whatever faith they are involved in. For some couples when one person is deeply involved in their faith-based practices, and the other one is not involved as much, this can be a source of tension for how to spend their free time. Even couples where both individuals are of the same faith, there can be differences in how they practice and the degree to which they practice. Sometimes spiritual advisers can help in teaching a couple how to navigate their differences and how to unify. I do not think religion should be a tool that divides, instead it can be used as an instrument that unifies through love and spiritual growth.

19. I want another child; my wife says one is enough. How do I convince her that our son would be better off with a sibling?

This is also a common scenario where one spouse wants more children than the other. Sometimes it is deciding between one or two, two or three, or greater than three children. The spouse who does not want more children may feel pressured and resent the other partner for trying to force the issue. Children can offer challenges like a more sizeable financial burden, less time with their partner, managing schedules, sleep disturbances, etc. However, many people also feel that the joys and rewards that come from raising children are well worth it. There can also be an issue of a woman feeling that she is running out of time and resenting her spouse for making her wait to have a child. If she is not successful later, she may resent her partner for wasting time.

It is important to express yourself and understand how sure you are of whether you do not want another child or whether you do. Also, it is useful to reflect on how big of a compromise would it be for you if your partner wants something different than you do. Sometimes issues around fertility can cause lots of tension in a relationship. Some therapists specialize in infertility and can help a couple express their feelings to each other to collectively arrive at a decision.

One of the challenges with big life dreams such as having or expanding a family, is that you see this being done with the cooperation of your partner, and you want them to support your dreams. There are increasing numbers of people becoming single parents by choice or leave relationships as they do not want to delay having a child. A common example of this is men who may want to take their time with committing or starting a family as they may feel there is no urgency to do so, and a woman may instead worry she is running out of time to achieve the goal of having her own family. If your partner is adamant in their position, sometimes there is not a whole lot you can do other than leaving the relationship to create space for other possibilities to occur with respect to family. Sometimes it may be futile to try and convince the other partner if they are fixated on their position and that may just be out of your control. Reconciliation with a partner even when you are not on the same page regarding having a family can be a painful and fretful journey, couples counseling may make this a bit more manageable.

20. Why does my daughter have night terrors?

Night terrors can happen in infants as young as 18 months. They take place during the first third of the night, during the deep non-dream sleep phase, otherwise known as non-REM sleep.[34] The infant may display behaviors, such as screaming, sweating, thrashing about, rapid breathing, open, glassy eyes, and a rapid heart rate. This can last anywhere from a few minutes to 45 minutes. The child will be able to fall back into a deep sleep and will not remember the episode. This is unlike a nightmare, where a child may become agitated or fearful the next morning when recalling the nightmare. Night terrors are thought to be due to overstimulation of the developing nervous system and they usually resolve over time.

One mother came to me quite frightened and upset about her three-year-old daughter, who, for about two months, had been waking up in the middle of the night screaming and thrashing about. "She seems awake," she told me, "but when I try to soothe her by holding her, it just gets worse. It is so scary to watch this and I do not know how to help her. The next morning, she seems to have no recall of what happened and doesn't seem bothered at all."

Even though this seems very scary to the mom, this can be a normal part of development and need not cause excessive concern. That said, you should contact your family pediatrician if you feel as if it might be something more than night terrors—like a seizure, when the entire body shake and a child may lose bowel or bladder control, bite his or her tongue. Night terrors can be exacerbated by poor sleep conditions and irregular sleep patterns. The American Academy of Pediatrics recommends that infants four to twelve months of age get 12 to 16 hours of sleep a day, including naps, and that infants ages one to two years of age get 11 to 14 hours of sleep a day. If you are having trouble establishing regular sleep patterns at home, it may be useful to work with a sleep consultant to assist in this area.

I recommend also looking at what is going on in your house. Is there too much ambient noise? Has your child been exposed to hours of electronic devices or lots of commotion in the house? Sensitive children can react poorly to certain stimuli, so take some time to evaluate the environment in your household and see what you can to ensure that it is mostly a calm, relaxing atmosphere.

21. My adopted son has a family history of bipolar disorder. Can I prevent him from developing the bipolar disorder?

According to studies in the US, about 25% of adults with bipolar disorder reported that they experienced their first episode of mania or depression before the age of 13, and 63-69% before the age of 19.[35,36,37] About 74% of children who have a parent with bipolar disorder develop a psychiatric disorder, with more than 20% having a diagnosis of either major depression, anxiety, ADHD, oppositional defiant disorder, and substance abuse.[38]

Bipolar disorder is a condition characterized by extreme changes in mood that can be potentially lifelong and cause functional limitations. In children experience symptoms of ADHD or irritability can be misdiagnosed with having bipolar disorder.[39] [40] This may lead to recommendations for certain treatments which are not clinically indicated or appropriate.

It is important that there be assessment of risk factors in children with family history of bipolar disorder or other mental illness. A history of adverse childhood experiences can increase the risk of earlier onset of mental illness like bipolar disorder and result in a more difficult course of illness.[41] Verbal abuse alone in the absence of physical or sexual abuse is also associated with an earlier onset of illness and more difficult course of bipolar disorder in adulthood.[42]

Psychosocial interventions can be effective and are low risk interventions. Family focused therapy (FFT) can be helpful with respect to disorders such as depression, bipolar disorder and prodromal (the period between the initial development of symptoms and presentation of illness) psychotic mental illness.[43]

If your child experiences mild anxiety, but not other symptoms, that risk factor can be addressed with cognitive behavioral therapy, positive lifestyle habits, and supplements that are in general regarded as safe. This are low risk interventions that can occur before considering medication management.[44] There is also research supporting the use of mindfulness-based cognitive therapy in children that are at risk for the development of bipolar disorder and are experiencing anxiety.[45] It is important to apply principles of what is considered generally good for child development such as music and sports programs that have a positive effect on the developing brain.[46] A child who has risk factors such as family history or is experiencing symptoms that maybe related to bipolar disorder could receive a more targeted and intensive approach.

22. My wife does not spend much time with my kids from a previous marriage. She acts annoyed when they are with us on visits. I feel she does not love them like she would if they were her own biological children. How do I deal with this?

The merging of any family can be stressful including and sometimes especially in blended families. It can be challenging for the children to have to navigate dealing with their parents' separation, having a new person enter their lives, and how to adjust to that new person. One of the misconceptions people have about marrying someone who does not have children is that they will automatically want to have the same type of relationship you do with your children. They may also be navigating their feelings of being an outsider trying to fit into a previously formed family. They may value their independence and may not quite be ready to be thrust into the role of co-parenting. The stepparent often has a difficult time defining their role, such as whether they are involved with discipline. It is a transition that may not occur seamlessly. They may be responsible at times for young children to keep them safe and a child or teenager may rebel against their disciplinary efforts.

Sometimes the stepparent introduces a lot of chaos into the family especially if they are abusive. Even without that, these events of emerging families can be still a challenge. Many blended families can work it out and develop a healthy dynamic. It is a matter of building effective communication, having healthy emotional boundaries, and mutual understanding. You may have to make peace with the fact that things may not start the way you imagined. The relationship your partner has with your children is a gradual growing relationship in the closeness can build over time. If it is not there right away, remember you are managing the emotions of different individuals including your children.

One of the biggest complaints of partners who enter relationships with people with children is that they do not get enough alone time with their partner and all the time ends up being family time. That may feel comfortable for you but not for your partner. If that is the case, then it is useful to set aside some time for date nights or options for the two of you to just connect. It is important to remember the other partner is not your children's parent, they are the stepparent, and their roles will be somewhat different than yours. This may be different if you are widowed where the stepparent plays a more prominent role in parenting in the absence of the other parent. Children may foster some feelings of resentment while still grieving the loss of their parent so need patience and empathy for them to develop comfort with the new person.

23. I try to avoid watching the news in front of my children usually but on occasion they have seen some content that is disturbing. How do I discuss some of the intense graphics and content they may happen to see?

It is wise to monitor the digital content your children receive. Studies after 9/11 showed that children who watched repeated footage of the events had symptoms of posttraumatic stress disorder.[47] The reality is media content has become more graphic and potentially traumatizing over the years. Studies have shown that African Americans, including children (particularly teenage boys), can experience symptoms of posttraumatic stress disorder watching repeated footage of police brutality.[48] The other danger is that for the white majority watching such footage, this can desensitize them towards acts of violence towards minorities, causing them to devalue the life of those of minority communities.[49,50]

Given that there is such an influx of digital content directed towards children it is useful to have some planning around this. There are current events shows curated specifically for children that can be appropriate. If they inadvertently watch graphic footage, you can have a discussion with them about it. Explaining that although some bad things happen in the world, we all can try to work together to prevent bad things from happening. Distracting them with more positive content can help divert their tension from ruminating on the disturbing content. It may be that you set aside time after they are asleep or when you can be away from them to watch the news. This may be a useful and exercise for you to also limit the amount of exposure you receive. Ultimately supervision around consumption, monitoring use, and limiting use and viewing of disturbing content can be protective for children.

24. My wife is very harsh with our daughter, yelling at her frequently. I do not think she will change any time soon. What can I do?

This can be difficult to watch, and you may battle feeling helpless that she will change. One way of intervening is having a firm conversation with your spouse about how this kind of behavior and interaction can be damaging to a child. Yelling out one time for your child to get out of the street when oncoming traffic is approaching is different than continuous yelling at home and reprimanding the child harshly with no positive reinforcement. Children can become anxious, stressed, have somatic complaints such as headaches and stomach aches, and other negative effects from verbal abuse. Verbal abuse can take the form of continuous yelling, using bad language, name-calling, harassment.

Sometimes a parent may just become flooded with intense emotion, especially in situations like your child is hitting another child or causing harm and that causes you to yell in frustration. You may find yourself yelling seeing harm happen to another person. Even still, it is good to sit down with your child and explain how that hurts another person and help them see the situation from that perspective. Seek to understand why they got angry and what ways you can help them manage their anger before they resort to aggression. You can discuss this approach with your wife as a better alternative. Setting up a reward system where a child receives a reward for keeping their hands to themselves can make parenting this behavior more positive and effective.

If your partner's behavior does not change, it is useful to suggest that your wife seeks the help of a therapist or you go to family therapy to address this. If she is not willing to go to a therapist, you can seek therapy to help you figure out the best way of addressing this. Sometimes a therapist may also view this behavior as abusive and outside intervention becomes involved such as with child protection services.

A woman who is under stress may take it out on her children, so one strategy may be mitigating her stress. Is she responsible for supporting the family? Is she responsible for working and household chores and other caretaking activities? Is she being mistreated by you or anyone in your family? One should never take out their anger towards a spouse on their children, but this happens a lot. Other factors may contribute to how a parent or spouse behaves.

When a person is going through a chronic medical illness or other life stressors, they may live in the space where they continuously take it out on their loved ones including their children. Understanding why that is happening can help you process your partner's behavior. Sometimes friends and family can intervene and explain things to your partner to help them change. If this behavior continues despite interventions, you may have to make the painful decision of whether to separate. Seeing this behavior repeatedly probably affects your feelings towards your spouse as well, causing fractures in the marital relationship. Separation does not also mean the behavior will stop, you may feel you have less ability to protect your daughter when she is with her mom and you are not, so that is also something to be dealt with. Your daughter should also have an individual therapist as this behavior may already be causing the formation of emotional scars that may affect her health long term.

25. My wife and I cannot get along. Is staying in a loveless marriage just as harmful to children as separating?

Marriage is an institution that has been dictated by societal norms and individual values. Many people believe that children do best in a healthy family network. Most professionals would agree this is best if the home environment is nurturing and safe. The issue of whether a parent puts their desires over a child's interest is a subject that is still being debated in religious circles, political platforms, and social media. Conservative religious groups that put a strong emphasis on the family network often counsel parents to work things out for the sake of their children. For political candidates, having a family and a spouse often helps their cause, as it may symbolize stability and commitment. Sometimes, people's belief in a faith keeps them committed to making their marriage work.

People who grew up in a family where their parents separated or divorced can be less surprised by being in a situation where they are considering the same path. Alternatively, coming from a broken home may also cause people to rush into trying to achieve domestic stability. Most parents tell me that splitting custody is one of the hardest parts of separation. It requires a gradual adjustment with a lot of support. If there was not a specific deal-breaker, such as abuse, addiction or adultery, some people may regret their decision years later. Addiction and adultery are things that people have worked through in marriage and managed to build trust again. If someone is in an abusive situation, whether they are the husband or the wife, psychological and physical damage can be inflicted on the victimized partner and their children. This can have all sorts of ramifications, such as increasing mental and physical illness, stress, and changes in a child's developing brain.[51] A decrease in anxiety after leaving an abusive situation can be restorative for yourself and your children.

Your wishes and freedom become intertwined with the needs of your children. It is important to be thoughtful and discerning about introducing new partners to your children, at any age. It is good to be aware of any red flags that may be potential issues concerning how your children will be treated. If you are not that serious with someone, it may cause pain in your children to develop a relationship with an adult who will end up leaving. Children may feel that you are betraying the other parent, even if you are no longer with them. They may act out and give your new partner a hard time. All these things are not surprising behaviors from children.

Many parents think that a toddler, for example, might not even remember their parents ever living together. It is possible that when a child is so young the adjustment can occur in a way where they do not have a memory of when their parents separated. There can be stress for the child as separation usually involves relocation and transitioning between two different environments. If there is no chance for marital issues to be resolved, then an amicable separation is the best way to handle it. It is not the conflict itself that predicts poor outcomes in children in the future, it is how the conflict is dealt with.

Marital counselors often include separation counseling as part of their services rendered to help with these transitions. The world is filled with different types of families, single-parent homes, LGBTQ families, etc. In some countries, the norm is for families to ebb and flow, to accept that sometimes things change, and it should not be feared.

I worked with a couple who had two children, both disabled. They were in an unhappy marriage for years but managed to get along with each other, mostly like roommates. Infidelity heightened their marital stress. After multiple discussions with me, as well as with individual and marital therapists, they decided that given their children's special needs and difficulty with any transitions, they would stay in the marriage until their children became adults. The parents then divorced and the children handled it gracefully. These parents felt this was the best decision for the sake of their children, but it was not easy for either of them to stay in the marriage. Talking to a trusted therapist about what you are going through can help you process your feelings and make decisions that work best for your family.

PART TWO

CHILDHOOD
6 TO 11 YEARS

1. No one invites my son to birthday parties, but his classmates will talk about going to each other's parties in school. This causes him to feel hurt and left out. What should I do?

Birthday parties may seem frivolous to some people, small occasions in the context of the many bigger problems we face on a day-to-day basis, but they can be a source of emotional stress in children and their parents. My parents did not usually celebrate my birthday in any big fashion. This may have been due in part to our culture, in India you are expected to treat others with presents instead of receiving things on your birthday. Growing up, I did not have birthday parties; nor was I allowed to attend most of my classmate's birthday parties. As a result, I did not even know if I was invited or not, so it did not seem relevant to me. In a way, this probably protected me from the heartache of not being invited to a particular child's birthday party and from having any specific expectations of what my birthdays should be like. My parents probably saved themselves a lot of stress this way, too. As an adult, I have come to enjoy rewarding myself a little on my birthday by mixing in some fun as I try to make it a spiritually uplifting time to celebrate myself and my life. It is understandable and a cultural norm to want to make a child feel special on their birthday and celebrate them in some way.

Sometimes it just hurts when a child is not invited to a party and for them, the reason often does not matter, children and adults yearn acceptance, fear rejection. It is important for your son to know that he is loved, especially when this type of rejection happens, and that he has qualities that make him lovable. Young kids do not understand that some of these things are just time-limited, and that elements like popularity often change during childhood and even in adulthood. If you can find a community that will embrace your family and incorporates fun activities for your son to do with others, he may be less focused on the pain of rejection.

Exposing him to cultural events, if you can find them in your area, can give him a sense of belonging. When your son becomes upset about not being invited, you can begin with a hug to comfort him and let him know that you love him unconditionally. At times, it is useful to talk with other parents about how you are feeling about your son being excluded. Parents have lots of different reasons for why they limit attendance at their child's party.

Sometimes, it is a numbers issue because of space and/or budget. Sometimes, they may prefer to avoid hosting a child who they feel might present a behavioral problem. Some parents may defer to their child choosing who comes and who does not. In some cases, parents opt to limit the number of guests because the birthday party can turn into an afternoon of unwelcome overstimulation for their child or due to recommended public health measures like those pertaining to COVID-19. In certain social circles, birthday parties ultimately became competitive events where parents try to upstage each other with how lavish and elaborate they can be. With COVID-19, gatherings for events like birthday parties have also been the cause of outbreaks, spreading the virus, and making it difficult to control the pandemic.

Remember that a child is much more likely to remember quality time with his friends and family. You can celebrate the day of their birth in so many economical ways that focus on people instead of things, which aim to bring children together as a group safely, even if it is virtually. Until the pandemic dies down, virtual gatherings are safest or socially distanced limited outdoor gatherings where mask-wearing is ensured. It can be useful to role model and remind your child that the quality of his daily relationships is more important than what happens one day of the year at a birthday party so that his expectations are not shattered if it is not perfect. Children can and should be excited about celebrating their day of birth, but it is important that they can internally appreciate and celebrate themselves on any day, which is ultimately emotionally self-empowering and does not depend on others' actions.

2. Should my daughter in first grade receive an allowance as an incentive for a good report card?

There are a lot of conflicting opinions among parents about the allowance issue. Some parents say they should not have to pay their kids for good behavior or good grades, but that should be just an expectation. Also, finances are an issue for so many families, so the priority of feeding a family and paying for essential expenses do not allow room for a monetary incentive for their children. There are creative ways to approach this so that an allowance does not have to mean financial payment necessarily.

A positive reinforcement system in the home can encourage more positive behaviors.[1] Children are individuals, not robots who come built to meet their parents' expectations and carry out all the tasks assigned to them. Some children do not offer resistance and follow through expectations but most often children will rebel against some things they are being told to do. This could be a result of how they are doing emotionally at that time or just not having a desire to do chores or lacking motivation or reacting to stress. Children who comply out of an unhealthy fear of their parents due to abuse leads to adverse health outcomes. With healthier family dynamics, fear of disappointing parents can result in a child's compliance as well, but this may be more out of respect for their parents as opposed to fear of harsh punitive actions.

Having an organized system that continually offers some reward for achieving goals or contributing to a household can be useful for children, to feel appreciated and motivated. It does not have to be in the form of a weekly payment. For young children it can be harder to stick to working towards a goal if the reward seems distant in the future. Rewards can be just spending some time with the child doing something they enjoy, taking them for an outing, indulging them with a treat, or other ways to make them feel good. This is not spoiling the child or setting up a situation where they do not develop their own internal drive. Parents are often better at taking things away than they are at giving a reward, so rewarding good behavior and ignoring bad behavior can be useful.

It is about simply offering them encouragement and appreciation. I do recommend that if the reward is monetary, it is good to also teach a child about how to manage money. How to save some of it, whether it is in a piggy bank or a bank account for an older child, learning how to allocate money to buy things, will help them learn to manage their own money. This is a useful skill for children to learn over time and not have to wait until they become an adult to build the skill set of learning to pay yourself first by investing in your future.

3. My son talks back to me a lot and uses swear words. Why does he act like this and what can I do about it?

Children can pick up certain habits from other family members and other kids they associate with. If they are around other children who talk back and use swear words, they may repeat that behavior. You may not be able to control everything that comes out of their mouth, but you can demand to be treated with respect. You can tell them if they use swear words or talk back significantly then they will not earn rewards for good behavior. Parents are often better at taking things away than they are at giving a reward, so rewarding good behavior and ignoring bad behavior can be useful.

I would also argue that you do not want to completely shut down efforts at self-assertion when they talk back, because sometimes children can be a good reflection on your behavior. If they have righteous anger about something such as how they are being treated or seeing others being treated poorly, and they talk back because of this, that is a good thing. They are learning to stand up to injustice. You want to be treated with respect and you will also want to encourage a process where children feel confident to assert themselves.

That is different from self-righteous anger, which involves a more primitive way of thinking such as talking back when appropriate limits are being put in place or making someone feel bad. Depending on their developmental age, children may not be able to discern the difference, in fact, a lot of adults have trouble discerning the difference between righteous and self-righteous anger. If the talking back and swearing continues, you can choose to just ignore it. Sometimes children are reacting to stress or difficult emotions and it may be useful to explore why this is happening as a way of helping them work through it. How you manage your own emotional reaction is important as children are often testing limits with their parents by acting out. If you also escalate your behaviors with along with them, it may just result in a dual escalation. Alternatively, if you disengage and do not reinforce the negative behavior with your negative behavior, the bad behavior does not have an audience.

4. My six-year-old son has a stuttering problem, which gets worse when he is asked to speak in front of people. How do I help him overcome this?

Stuttering is not uncommon. Sometimes children develop stuttering when they are dealing with anxiety from stress at home or independently have anxiety related to stuttering.[2]

Stuttering is a speech impediment that can have genetic origins. Getting an evaluation with a speech therapist can be helpful and regular speech therapy can help address the issue.

Bolstering self-esteem with therapy and teaching a child to learn to manage anxiety may also help deal with anxiety-provoking situations such as speaking in public or socially which may increase stuttering.[3] Stuttering can wax and wane throughout a lifetime so if it looks like your child overcame it but then it returned do not be disheartened. It may require just a return to some of the previous interventions. Methods used in speech therapy or other interventions need to be practiced, and with any acquired skill set sometimes your skills get rusty and you need a reminder. You can tell your child it is like learning a new instrument, sometimes it is important to continue practicing so you get better and better at it. The important thing is for them not to feel ashamed about it.

It is helpful to communicate with their teachers and make sure teachers understand how to be patient with your child. They should be careful to not rush the child or forcefully try to change this habit. The speech therapist can also work with the school on this. There are many successful people and renowned public speakers who have dealt with stuttering and learn to overcome it. President Joe Biden has dealt with stuttering and has been open about discussing his challenges. You can tell your child that sometimes the things we consider to be weaknesses can become our source of strength. Having to deal with a challenge like stuttering can help you become more compassionate towards other people who are struggling, increase your patience with others and yourself.

It can also be an opportunity to teach your child the importance of self-compassion and forgiving himself or herself for not being perfect as no one is. These are powerful, useful skills that it will serve your child well. So instead of looking at stuttering as an insurmountable challenge, you can teach your child to view it as an opportunity for growth. There are also organizations like the International Stuttering Association that provide resources and avenues for support such as support groups for those who deal with this challenge. When I meet a child patient who has an issue with stuttering, I still speak to them as if we are having a regular conversation. When they stumble on a word or begin to stutter, I remind myself to just wait patiently and allow the child to work through the process. This patience is so vital because a child needs to know that you will just be present when they are confronted with difficulty. Do not rush them, do not shame them, and be gentle in how you approach stuttering. It will ultimately serve your child well to feel nurtured while dealing with this.

5. My seven-year-old son has difficulty reading compared to his peers. How can I help him improve at reading?

Children learn to read at different speeds. There are many reasons why one child may not be able to pick up reading as fast as another. There are some possibilities worth knowing about, which may need to be explored as you confer with your son's teacher and doctor.

Stress can affect a child's ability to focus and learn. Is your home environment traumatic or toxic? Abuse in the home, domestic violence, or parents or siblings dealing with substance issues can cause stress. Even dealing with health issues of family members can be a source of stress on a child. Although some stresses cannot be erased, such as if you have an elderly grandparent dealing with health issues living in the house, you can help a child navigate their emotions and feel encouraged to read. Any sort of abusive environment must be corrected because the longer that persists the worse it is for a child's mental health.

Hearing loss is sometimes not detected early enough. Children who have had multiple ear infections may be at risk for hearing loss, sometimes temporarily, but it can be enough to affect their ability to learn and speak, which is vital to read. Audiology testing can help screen for hearing deficits, which then can be addressed with hearing aids or other modalities such as cochlear implants.

Too much screen time can be a source of overstimulation, which distracts a child from being able to focus on reading, and this exposure should be limited. Visual problems, which can be corrected with proper eyewear, can create visual deficits that make it hard to read. A vision evaluation can reveal the need for corrective glasses. Sometimes, a child may have undiagnosed dyslexia. Many celebrities have disclosed struggling with dyslexia as young children, feeling marginalized and incompetent from their disability. If this is identified, there are accommodations to help a child read.

Some children may have auditory or visual processing deficits that make it hard for them to absorb what they are looking at on a page. There are specific psychoeducational evaluations that can evaluate for these processing deficits. If they do exist, schools can put in place certain accommodations to help a child overcome these deficits to become a better reader. Mental health issues, such as ADHD, depression, anxiety, and Autism Spectrum Disorder can interfere with a child's ability to focus, absorb, and read. Teachers and parents can fill out rating scales as part of the assessment in evaluating whether your child is dealing with any of these issues.

Medical issues, such as anemia or a thyroid imbalance, can affect concentration and the ability to focus on reading. These can be ruled out by a pediatrician. Micronutrient deficiencies in the diet can also influence a child's medical and mental health, which in turn can affect their reading. No matter what issues your child may be facing, reading to him has benefits. It can help him relax into a restorative wind down routine, encourages bonding, and it will allow him to become increasingly familiar with the spoken word. I have fond memories of my father taking us to the library. He loved to read and transmitted that same passion to his children, a love of books. If your child sees you reading it may increase their curiosity to do so.

Over the summer, I often inquire whether my child patients have been reading, particularly those in urban environments and those living in unsafe neighborhoods without easy access to a library. I ask them if they have books in their home and if they do not, I help the parents figure out a way to access reading materials. Teaching your child to enjoy reading can help them perform better in school, both short-term and long-term. Holidays offer a great opportunity to encourage reading for fun. If your son or daughter is struggling to read, do not hesitate to ask your child's teacher and school administration for assistance on how to improve. Public school districts in the U.S. use what are called Individual Education Plans (IEP) that can be implemented for children who are struggling with any of the conditions covered here.

6. My eight-year-old daughter wants to join gymnastics. I am hesitant to commit to having to drive her around to several practices a week plus tournaments, which is what this gymnastics studio requires. How do I support her, encourage exercise, but respect my time as well?

Children and adults should stay physically active. It is important to cultivate from a young age a lifestyle that is not sedentary and incorporates physical activity. Getting involved in sports is a great way for children to get physical activity, learn pro-social skills such as teamwork and sportsmanship. However, for many parents, including single parents and working parents, it can be hard to logistically be available for all their children's practices and games. During the COVID-19, team sports have been limited for many children to prevent spread of the virus, which also limits structured exercise.

It can also be financially difficult as many recreational sports teams in the community often require payment for coaching and fatigue on the part of the parents for having to be responsible for making sure your child gets to their practices. Sports at schools particularly the high school level in the west can be competitive. If the child does not have a head start on athletic skill-building, it can be hard to pick up and play at the same level as some of her classmates.

I believe that if children show interest in the sport they should be allowed to participate, and it should not be limited to those who just show aptitude. This is because it just further perpetuates the problem of a child who has not had exposure to that physical activity not getting more exposure. In communities where there is a lot of driving involved to take children to some of these group activities, parents can feel exhausted and stressed having the responsibility of shuttling their children around.

There are some ways to reduce your sense of exhaustion. One is participating in carpools which may have to wait during the COVID-19 pandemic until it safe to do so. Choosing one or two activities you want your children to be involved in can help keep a manageable schedule. Gymnastics can help with strength building, balance, and cardio activity. It can also build a child's self-esteem if they begin to feel better as their skills advanced. The downside of gymnastics, especially competitive gymnastics, is that there is a risk of injuries, stress on joints, even a possible reduction in height.[4][5][6][7][8][9] This also can depend on how much your child practices and for how long. It is important to note that there can be a risk of injury with many sports as well. If you are worried about some things specific to gymnastics, choosing other sports for your child to be involved in can be just as fulfilling for her. Also finding instructors who are mindful of injury prevention and not pressuring a child to push themselves while injured is important.

The other thing that happens is sometimes when parents are busy taking their children to different activities, they can neglect their own physical health. It is important that you also pay attention to your need for physical activity. If it means going for a walk while your child is at practice, lifting some light weights at home, or any other way like you can keep yourself physically active even in short intervals, this is beneficial for you. Children being involved in sports can also be motivating for adults. I have known of parents who also start taking an adult dance class motivated by their children dancing. This can be an opportunity for you to utilize the beauty of the human body with movement.

7. My Hispanic eight-year-old daughter came home crying one day, saying she wanted blonde hair and blue eyes like some of her classmates. How do I explain to her that her uniqueness is beautiful?

Children are so often the recipients of subtle and not-so-subtle messages of racial bias, and it has an impact. This may be with respect to skin color, hair color, or eye color. Even in countries where the race is mostly the same, colorism takes place, where preference is given to lighter skin complexion. This belief system descends from the original colonizer mentality. This perpetuated preferential attitude results in girls and women feeling unattractive, spending money on lightening creams and other products to make them look more fair-skinned. Studies have even shown that young children may attribute more positive qualities to lighter skin than darker skin.[10] Excessive lavishing praise of physical attributes makes cultivate narcissistic tendencies which is much different than building self-esteem.

You can facilitate dialogue and explore out of curiosity about why she is thinking that way? You can challenge her beliefs by asking her if looking different is a bad thing, and if she believes that, then why? I remember having some of these thoughts myself when I was younger. They are not always negative in nature, sometimes it can just be a curiosity factor of what it would be like to look different. A short person may want to know what it feels like to be tall and vice versa. The problem is when there are negative attributes associated with one feature and positive attributes associated with others.

However, we are now seeing ads in the media embracing diversity in the realms of skincare, make-up, clothing, etc. The more diversity is represented in society, the more welcoming a child may feel.

This may be hard to do if you are in an area where there is not a lot of diversity. This may mean you have to make extra effort to make sure your child feels good about themselves for their differences. Having your child meet with a culturally competent therapist can be helpful to build her self-esteem.

8. My daughter saw a man expose himself on the street. How do I talk to her about what he did?

There are so many things that we wish we could shield our children from, such as indecent exposure. Some situations are unfortunately unavoidable. It is not socially acceptable to disrobe in public in many societies. In some regions and villages in different parts of the world, this may not be a big deal and children may be used to seeing this. You can talk to her about how she felt seeing that and explore what made her fearful. You can explain to her that sometimes there are people who struggle with things in their head, and they engage in behaviors without understanding the consequences. You do not want your child to blur the boundaries between appropriate adult behavior towards her or not appropriate behavior.

This can be a good opportunity to discuss the difference between good touch and bad touch. You can explain that if something happens that makes her feel uncomfortable, she should feel comfortable coming to you or another trusted adult to talk about it. You do not have to talk about the incident repeatedly, but if you put it into context at a developmentally appropriate age, you can help your child process it and move in without being traumatized. It is also useful to reassure your child that you are there to protect her and keep her safe. Distraction can be useful if she seems to get stuck on what she saw. Showing some signs of fear soon after, worrying about seeing the man again, are not uncommon, but if these symptoms continue to persist, you may want to seek therapy for her.

9. My father-in-law uses inappropriate and foul language around my children. My wife wants him to be in our lives, but I do not want our children being exposed to this. How do I handle this?

It is become more culturally acceptable to use inappropriate language and profanity in certain families, and communities. Children may be getting exposure from classmates and other sources, but it is understandable to want to limit this kind of exposure. The first step would be to have your wife have a conversation with her father about amending this behavior around the kids. You might want to have this conversation as well with him. Explain that you do not want your children to be exposed to this kind of language and you do not want to hear it come from him. If he is dismissive and refuses to change which is a possibility, then you may have to change your strategy.

Sometimes when there are problematic family members such certain in-laws, you may have to limit interactions and have boundaries. It is good to have a conversation with your wife about how she feels about what is happening. She may be so used to his behavior that it is not jarring for her because it is the norm. You might have to have in place a strategy and let your father-in-law know that if he starts using inappropriate language, you will have to leave with your children. It would also be good to have a conversation with your children. You do not need to put down your father-in-law, but you can discuss with your children that you do not like some of the language that is used, and you are trying to encourage him to change. With certain individuals getting into heated arguments may only increase the behavior you are trying to make them stop doing. Some individuals are not people you can talk to as they cannot self-reflect and show empathy for those they are affecting. In this case, external limits and boundaries must be implemented and adhered to.

10. My 10-year-old daughter has lots of anxiety on planes. How do I prepare her for flights?

Anxiety is a common childhood condition. According to the Centers for Disease Control and Prevention, 7.1% It is estimated that between the ages of three and 17 have a diagnosed anxiety. The best way to address the issue of anxiety is preparation. Anxiety can happen when there is environmental stress. For example, if there is a lot of loud arguing in your house, that may contribute to a child developing anxiety. Sometimes, anxiety is situational. For example, this girl only has anxiety on planes. The first step in dealing with this involves having a conversation with her, asking what it is about flying that specifically makes her scared.

It could be the sound of the engine during takeoff or the sensation in her stomach as the plane rises in the air. It could be from the newness of the experience. It helps to offer reassurance that there is a lot of work that goes into making sure that a plane is safe to take off with passengers. Children can develop anxiety if they see news of a plane crash. The tragedy of 9/11 caused great anxiety in children (and adults) when footage of the plane attacks aired non-stop on TV throughout the day and night. One way of helping a child become comfortable with planes is to engage in play. You can imitate what a takeoff looks like with a toy plane or paper airplane to simulate the experience.

Deep breathing exercises and progressive muscle relaxation techniques can help children combat anxiety. There are many online and book resources to help you teach these techniques. A licensed and trained therapist can teach and repeat these techniques with the child. Sometimes, carrying a transitional object along, like a stuffed animal or favorite blanket, can help with flight anxiety. Having fun things to do on the plane, such as a coloring book, can be a good source of distraction. Melatonin taken before a flight can relieve anxiety and help relax a child, but that is to be discussed with your child's doctor. For severe anxiety, talking to your child's pediatrician or child psychiatrist about medication management for situational anxiety can be an option.

11. We just moved into a largely Caucasian community and my ten-year old son is getting bullied at school. How do I protect him?

Micro and macro aggressions can be considered as forms of bullying. It can result in anxiety, diminish self-esteem, depression, and other effects on mental health.[11] [12] This means that it is important to address these things as it can result in a lot of pain and affect mental health even later in life. I still remember how painful it was to be bullied and have experienced being on the receiving end of micro and macroaggressions. This is a systemic issue end it is important to address this with leadership at the school. Unfortunately, often those in leadership positions do not either want to acknowledge a problem, do not think it is a problem, or are in denial. In the US, there was a viral video of a student forced to cut his dreadlocks if he wanted to participate in a wrestling match. This caused a lot of outrage and conversation about hair discrimination. Most if not all black parents in western society have "the talk" with their black sons regarding how to interact with the police. Parents do this because they know their son can be the victim of racial profiling and police brutality. It is so important to fill your child up with positivity and a healthy self-image. It is imperative that bullying is addressed so that it does not continue and cause mental health issues. A culturally competent therapist can help him process what happened and how to build resilience from it.

12. I have three children, ages six, eight, and nine. How much social media is okay for them?

The American Academy of Pediatrics recommends no digital screen time for the first two years of life, with exception of video chatting with family members and family friends. Over the age of two, the recommendation is no more than two hours of screen time a day.

Because of the COVID-19 pandemic and virtual schooling, children are spending more and more time in front of screens. Children often do a lot of their school assignments online as well, so it is hard to limit use. They do need to take breaks from staring at the screen as it can cause eye strain, poor posture, and other health effects. Using dictating software can sometimes help avert eyes away from the screen at times. Encouraging children to read books and using screen time apart from schoolwork as a reward on occasion instead of continuous use, can be useful in limiting use to some degree. If the TV is on all the time in the home, that is what children are going to be exposed to, so it is important for the parents to also will model limiting screen time. This can be hard to do because for many professions that are not manual labor work, they involve the use of digital technology as well. Taking breaks from it is vital for our health and children's health. Taking walks together as a family, playing interactive games, allowing children to use their imagination to play, can help get children and well as parents away from screen time. Creativity and the use of imagination are especially important for the development and growth of children.

13. My husband told our 10-year-old son that men do not cry. I think this is harmful and will prohibit our son from expressing himself. How do I make my husband understand?

Gender defined roles and attributes have been ascribed to men and women over time, passed on from generation to generation. Not allowing a child to express themselves when feeling emotions of sadness or other emotions may prohibit needed emotional healing. They may instead take out their feelings on others and it can affect their mental health. Recognizing one's emotions and learning appropriate ways of expressing them is an important aspect of social development. Having pent-up emotions is not great for our immunity and it is not great for our well-being in general, physically, or mentally. When a child expresses himself or herself, he or she can be educated about how to deal with emotions constructively in an empathic fashion. Not knowing what your child is feeling can be detrimental to the child. So many stories from families of children who have committed suicide show that a lot of the time parents are not even aware of how much their child is suffering.

There is an element of teaching children to regulate their emotions so that the expression does not become detrimental to them. In adulthood, some people can cry or become emotional every time someone gives them constructive criticism. This becomes a defense mechanism where they deflect the attention from their behaviors. The same dynamic happens sometimes during difficult discussions on race or other interpersonal dynamics. This also often happens in the workplace when allegations of racism or sexism happen, there is defensiveness and anger about being labelled as racist or sexist.

There also is a phenomenon where one gets emotional about an injustice that does not exist. This can be hard to tease out because one may feel they are passed up for a promotion because they are a woman, because of race, or because of religious preferences. The tricky part here is that all of that can be true and all of that can also be denied as contributing factors by the other party, making it hard to prove. Figuring out constructive ways to manage your emotions when dealing with these themes can be useful. It is important not to feel disempowered but to feel strong. We want young boys to grow up to be empathetic, strong, compassionate, and in touch with their emotions. It is healthy to cry when you suffer a loss and grieve appropriately. Learning not to cry every time you do not get a toy that you want may help develop a constructive path in dealing with life's disappointments. Not breaking down in tears when someone brings up an action that has been perceived to be insensitive by you can also be useful in acknowledging the truth and acting for correction. The aim is to improve self-reflection and self-correction in the context of emotional growth.

14. I recently heard my 11-year-old daughter making fun of another child with her friends. How do I teach empathy and teach my child not to become a bully?

One of the best ways to do this is by role modeling. There is a difference between joking in jest to generate laughter and doing it at someone else's expense. Even as adults we are sometimes unaware that playful teasing may be hurtful. Having several conversations about treating other people with fairness and kindness should be part of an ongoing family discussion. Children will imitate what their parents do so if they see their parents viciously gossiping about others repeatedly then they may pick up that habit. No one is perfect and sometimes we may indulge in these behaviors without realizing that the children are listening. The first step as a parent is committing to your own self-reflection. Notice if you are engaging in these behaviors and take measures to correct them.

You can also explain to children that the effects of bullying can affect someone throughout their life, and you do not want other children to become traumatized in this way. Having an honest, open discussion is much more useful than yelling at them. Ask your child why they felt they needed to engage in this behavior, was it a matter of fitting in with their friends? Did they feel that if they did not also participate in making fun of someone they would be shunned by their peers? If so, why is that? Why are those friendships so important anyways if it means you can only be a friend if you participate in bullying behaviors?

Most children and even adults would rather be part of the safe majority than be the one who gets picked on. However, it is also important to teach children that sometimes being unpopular by standing up for right versus wrong is much more admirable in the long run. A good exercise is role-playing. Role modeling how to stand up for someone being bullied can help them want to do that in the future. Engaging in a discussion of what it must feel like to be bullied is also useful. Even as adults, we must learn to draw hard boundaries when we experience bullying behavior, and we must be mindful that we do not fall into a group dynamic such as what we see in certain smear campaigning political arenas. We must teach children to understand another person's feelings and develop the skills of setting appropriate boundaries while also learning about the benefits of an emotionally generous heart. Those of religious faith can share stories in scriptures of morality and caring about others, a common theme in most religious faiths.

15. As a minority parent, I am worried about if my kids, ages 11 and 13, will be able to grow up in such a prejudiced society and appreciate the value of who they are. What are the effects of racial trauma and bias on my children's mental health?

The American Academy of Pediatrics has issued a policy statement on the impact of racism on child and adolescent health. While there has been some historical progress toward establishing racial equality and equity, there is a negative ongoing impact of racism on health, including the health of children.[13] The first step in addressing this is raising awareness that it is an issue. Just because legalized slavery and separate but equal water fountains and bathrooms have been abolished as standard practice, does not mean that the perpetual stress of racism is not putting people at an unfair disadvantage based on their race.

We know that a child's environment should be nurturing and loving. Treatment that chips away at this optimal setting can be damaging to a child's mental health. Several studies show that racism is been a big driver of healthcare inequality.[14] One dark example of this is the disparity in maternal health care.[15] In the US, black women are less likely to receive correct diagnoses of conditions, such as endometriosis, and pain reported by black women is not taken as seriously compared to white women.[16] As a result, it can go undertreated and can lead to long-lasting health consequences. Medical research has typically excluded diverse groups and under-represented minorities.[17] This has resulted in flawed science, justifying differential treatment.

Modern science shows that humans are 99.9 percent the same at the level of their genome.[18] Children can distinguish physical differences concerning race beginning in infancy. As they grow, they become inoculated with explicit and implicit biases transmitted from their environment and families of origin. In many nations, children experience structural racism based on where they live, where they get an education, their parent's economic status, and how the law values their human rights. Research shows that a positive racial identity provides for more optimal development. This is particularly critical during adolescence. Even child bystanders who witness acts of racism can be affected in negative ways. A child who experiences racism can internalize negative stereotypes about himself or herself.

If a child is told repeatedly by peers, teachers, and society in general that people who look like them do not get a higher education and do not have skills that allow them to succeed vocationally and professionally, they may grow up to play out that stereotype. Even though federal civil rights laws prohibit discrimination, more African American and Native American students in the US get suspended from school than white children.[19] African American children get expelled almost twice as much as white students.[20] Racism can cause physiological changes in a child's body, including a rise in stress hormones, anxiety, depression, poor self-esteem, and lack of motivation.[21] [22] Racism is a type of trauma for the victim, and trauma can cause structural changes in the brain, some of which may be irreversible.[23]

More recently we have seen evidence of racial inequality on a national stage with children being separated from families at the US/Mexican border and put in cages. This is willful causation of unnecessary trauma and stress in these children that can have long-lasting effects. This kind of trauma can put a child at risk for acquiring numerous medical illnesses and mental health issues.[24]

It is important to work with your child's school to make sure that he or she has access to supportive education that fights against institutional racism. It is important to speak out when you see racism or discrimination and encourage your child to do so as well. We need to communicate with children about this and teach them healthier ways to view themselves and each other regardless of racial or ethnic background. Poverty and racism often exist together, so it is also important that we participate in programs that help lift people out of poverty.

16. My 11-year-old son does not want to talk to our family. He just goes into his room and listens to music or watches videos. How do I get him to engage with the family?

When children enter their teenage years, they progress into a phase that has been described by Erickson's theory of psychological development as identity versus role confusion. As children grow, they feel more connected to their peers and begin to see themselves as separate thinking individuals from their family members, with their own beliefs and ideas. One of the problems with digital technology is that the addictive nature as it has taken the place of a lot of natural organic social interaction. Listening to music can be a relaxing coping mechanism for young people. It is important to distinguish whether your child is isolating because they are depressed or because they just do not feel like interacting as much with their family due to a desire for more independence.

If interactions are contentious and a teen receives a lot of reprimanding about school performance or chores, he or she may choose to isolate and not interact to avoid negative interactions. Self-reflection without judgement can sometimes give you a more objective view of things. Is there anything that you could be transferring in your interaction with your children that may them not want to open? Limiting technology use may allow for more social interaction with the family. Having rituals like eating meals together as a family can also be useful to improve social interaction. If your child engages well with peers, is not involved in any self-destructive behavior, and is functioning well overall, this also may be a phase that improves with time. Again, asking your child if they would like to talk to someone on the outside like a therapist may help them disclose discomfort or uncover certain issues.

17. We live in a disenfranchised neighborhood that has significant amounts of crime. What should we tell our two boys about gun violence?

Unfortunately, this is often a conversation that for African American parents in the US cannot avoid especially when it comes to police interactions. There has been a disproportionate number of police brutality incidents that have resulted in the loss of life of African Americans.[25] Gun violence does exist all over the world and in some places, it is much more prevalent. Engaging in discussions about gory details is not helpful and may only frighten children. Having a frank discussion about how guns can be extremely dangerous is useful, however. Speaking in generalities like telling your child that you want to watch them when they are playing to make sure that they are safe is a good way to present the topic. This is especially relevant if you live in an area with much gun violence and must increase your vigilance around your child's safety.

Children can get scared when they see law enforcement with guns. Letting them know that these individuals carry guns to protect people from bad guys and that there are a lot of good people who serve in law enforcement can help balance anxiety. It is important to tell children not to touch guns unless it is the sheer act of self-defense where they are able to knock a gun out of a perpetrator's hand or remove it from someone's reach such as another young child. Unfortunately, many schools have had to have shooter drills where children are taught to hide in the closet with their teacher or under their desks in case a shooter entered the school.

It is responsible to tell children that guns can really hurt or even kill, so our children should stay away from them. If you live in a neighborhood where there is active and frequent gun violence, you may have to be very hypervigilant as a parent for the survival of your family. This is a reality for so many living in areas of battling religious and political factions. It may mean spending more time indoors which of course should not have to be a necessity for a child who needs nature and fresh air but may be required. Teaching them safety skills such as what to do if they hear what sounds like gunshots can help them build potential lifesaving thought processes.

Many children live in violent neighborhoods but are not aware of the violence that is around them because they are sheltered by the protective forces of their family and others. The adults in the family may work together to keep the home environment joyous and upbeat so the children feel safe. Many of these children can grow up without being traumatized. Of course, if given the option most families would want to escape from threats of gun violence but so often circumstances do not allow for that. So many families have pleaded worldwide to seek refuge to escape from gun violence only to receive more trauma by harsh immigration policies post-migration such as the US/Mexican border. As a parent, it may help to get involved in anti-gun violence campaigns and initiatives to increase the safety of children.

18. My children feel bad that we cannot afford certain things that their friends have. How do I discuss class differences with my children?

When children enter their teenage years, they progress into a phase that has been described by Erikson's theory of psychological development as identity versus role confusion. As children grow, they feel more connected to their peers and begin to see themselves as separate thinking individuals from their family members, with their ideas and beliefs. One of the problems with digital technology is that the addictive nature as it has taken the place of a lot of natural organic social interaction. Listening to music can be a relaxing coping mechanism for young people.

It is important to distinguish between if your child is isolating because they are depressed, or they just do not feel like interacting as much with their family. If interactions are contentious and a teen feels they are being reprimanded frequently about school performance, he or she may choose to isolate to avoid the interaction. Self-reflection in a way free of self-judgement may give a more objective view of your interaction with your child. Is there anything that you are saying or doing that may potentially make your child feel uncomfortable feelings? Is there a way to hold them accountable for things like school and chores but still allow for enjoyment so they feel rewarded? These things may help a teen want to interact more with family.

Limiting technology used may allow for more social interaction with family. Having rituals like eating meals together as a family can also be useful to improve social interaction. If your child engages well with peers, is not involved in any self-destructive behavior, and is functioning well overall, this also may be a phase that improves with time. Asking your child if they would like to talk to someone on the outside like a therapist may help them disclose discomfort or uncover certain issues.

19. My son has expressed suicidal thoughts. Why is this happening and how do I know if he is serious about acting on these thoughts?

A young person having suicidal thoughts is something that needs immediate attention. Teenagers can be impulsive and not be able to think of possible positive outcomes in the future when they are faced with moments of desperation. Suicidal thoughts can occur with symptoms of depression. If your son seems sad or irritable much of time, does not seem to enjoy himself, lacks motivation, has trouble concentrating, these can all signify the presence of depression. If he feels guilt, has sleep and appetite disturbances, has low energy or fatigue, these are also possible symptoms of depression.

When I hear about something like this, one of the first things to do is make sure he does not have access to things he can use to hurt himself, such as firearms, pill bottles, knives, etc. If a young person is feeling this way, they should have been supervised to prevent acting on impulses and evaluation by a trained mental health professional who knows how to address suicidal ideation. He may require outpatient treatment, or inpatient treatment for stabilization if his thoughts are intrusive and he thinks of carrying out a plan. This is for the trained mental health professional to decide and guide you through the process of next steps. What you do not want to do is respond to this with judgment, sarcasm, criticism. Saying things like "get over it," "Do it if you are serious," "don't be so weak," are not supportive and may contribute to reinforcing the will to act on it.

I have met too many parents who have had to deal with the loss of a child due to suicide and it brings about incredible pain and so many of them suffer from guilt that they could not prevent it. This may be a window of opportunity for you to get your son the help that he requires. Suicidal ideation is something that should be taken seriously, even if you do not believe he is serious. As a parent, you cannot be completely objective, and your son may not even disclose to you if he has a plan or the seriousness of his ideation. When we encounter stressful moments in life, we may have thoughts of not wanting to be around as a reflection of feeling helpless or hopeless, but if these thoughts are more than fleeting, and there is a fixation on not wanting to be alive, this can become a potentially fatal scenario.

Teen suicide is the second leading cause of death among adolescents in the US.[26] In addition, using substances can increase the risk of suicide attempts.[27] A skilled therapist can help build your son's coping skills so that he does not spiral down into having these thoughts and learn to reach out for help if he does confront them. You do not want to dismiss this language if you hear from your son that he is entertaining these thoughts. It is okay as a parent to check in now and then with your child if they are having any dark thoughts about life.

There are many educational materials online about teen suicide and many countries have hotline numbers that teens can call if they are experiencing these thoughts. Please invest in the due diligence to find out what is available in your area and make sure your teen has access to those numbers in case he experiences troubling thoughts such as these. Sometimes these thoughts are time-limited during a stressful time and they go away, but sometimes they persist, and more severe mental illness needs to be ruled out. Fortunately, now there are more treatments available to help manage depression and if teens are permitted access to the appropriate resources, they can find a support system to help them cope with these thoughts.

20. My 12-year-old daughter has been steadily gaining weight. The doctor says that according to her body mass index (BMI) she is overweight for her height. How do I encourage a healthy diet and lifestyle without making her feel bad about her body image?

Healthy lifestyles, weight management, and body image are issues that affect so many families. According to the American Academy of Child and Adolescent Psychiatry (AACAP), approximately 12.7 million, or 17 percent of children and adolescents in the United States, are obese. According to the World Health Organization, in 2016 an estimated 340 million children and adolescents between the ages of 5-19 were overweight or obese, and in 2019, an estimated 32.8 million children under the age of five were considered overweight or obese. The Center for Disease Control defines overweight by the criteria of a Body Mass Index (BMI) at or above 85th percentile, and a child is considered obese if the BMI is above the 95th percentile in comparison to children and teens the same age and sex.

If a child is obese during adolescence, studies show that they have an 80 percent chance of remaining obese as an adult.[28] Many causes contribute to obesity, starting with family history. If one parent is obese, their child has a 50 percent chance of becoming obese. When both parents are obese, chances go up to 80 percent.[29][30] Certain medical problems can contribute to obesity, but it is usually caused by other factors, including genetics, activity level, psychological, and environmental factors.[31] Stressful life events, stress within the family, low self-esteem, and emotional problems, such as depression can also cause obesity. Many risks and complications are associated with obesity, such as an increased risk of heart disease, high blood pressure, diabetes, trouble sleeping, high cholesterol, and joint pain.[32][33]

Some ways to assist in weight loss include dietary changes such as avoidance of sugary drinks and encouraging physical activity.[34] It is important to maintain a child's self-esteem while implementing a weight management program in the home. Praising healthy habits, such as exercise and healthy eating, can help motivate a child, as well as a reward system for maintaining healthy habits. It is always important to reassure your daughter that she is loved by you regardless, that she is worthwhile, and it is what is on the inside that matters most. When she questions why she cannot have more food or junk food, you can respond by saying that doctors have instructed families to adopt healthy lifestyles together, which means eating better and making smarter choices.

If you eliminate most junk food in the house, serve snacks, such as fresh fruit and nuts instead of processed foods, over time a child can learn to reach for these better options when she has a hunger pang. Parents often do not realize that typical juices contain a lot of sugar and can contribute to weight gain. The same is true with sodas. Sparkling water can be a good substitute for children to transition them off soda or in place of soda. Encouraging fresh fruit over juices can also help. Of course, dark green vegetables, such as spinach, broccoli, and kale, are healthy options.

If you continue to focus on being healthy and stay away from highlighting body image and attraction, that will help keep your daughter's self-esteem at a healthy high level. We owe it to the next generation to try and protect self-esteem without encouraging any narcissistic self-imaging. Children and adults should not feel that they are worse than others, and but also not feel they are better than everyone. It is ultimately better for a child's self-esteem if you praise their effort. For example, if they are working hard on a school project, you can praise the effort as opposed to praising them for being "smart." This is because praising things that are not in their control may cause them to not feel they have the agency to create a new reality based on discipline and motivation. You can tell your daughter that she is beautiful to you because you think she simply is a beautiful human being. Teaching her to appreciate and cultivate qualities that will help her develop compassion for herself and others will help her not feel dependent on physical qualities. Encouraging your daughter to feel good about herself because of her uniqueness and embrace her worth even while trying to achieve certain health related goals can make the obsession around image less prominent.

21. What is the best way to advocate for my disabled child?

Having a child with a disability can provide additional challenges with respect to parenting and addressing that your child's special needs are met. Many parents experience grief witnessing their child struggle with certain medical and mental health issues, anxiety about the future and their child's prognosis, concerns about getting the proper treatment, and medication related concerns. All of this takes an enormous psychological toll on a parent or parents. Sometimes the stress also causes difficulty with co-parenting especially when there is disagreement on the approach and type of treatment. Some parents can be in denial or not want to confront the reality of the situation. Many parents feel very guilty that they did not do enough to prevent the disability or address it early enough. Women can experience feeling guilty that they did not take care of themselves well enough during pregnancy or whether it was a result of something else like not breastfeeding, that resulted in their child's disability.

There can be a huge amount of multitasking that often comes into play, scheduling different doctor's appointments and other interventional treatments, making sure medication is available and accessible, addressing side effects from medication, navigating educational systems, transportation issues, financial stresses, etc. There also exists variability of available resources in different parts of the world. Wheelchair accessibility is one such issue that limits the ability of disabled people to be able to participate in both functional and leisure activities.

Housing challenges are also problematic for so many families with disabled children or adults, finding dwellings that are handicap accessible, have elevators, etc. Caregiving needs may not be covered completely or at all by insurance. Parents may also feel that any caregiving that they are given may not be sufficient for their child's needs and they also feel if they do not do it, something important will be missed. There may need to be attention to things like catheter changes in children with paralysis, diaper changes and prevention of bedsores, administration of in-home dialysis in those with kidney failure.

Caregivers need support and they need breaks for their emotional and physical health as well. It is important to be mindful of how that can be attended to within the context of advocacy efforts. It is important to advocate for your child and yourself. The first step with advocacy involves gathering information. Making sure your child receives medical and mental health care as needed, understanding their diagnosis, collaborating with different entities regarding treatment planning and what treatments are required, and what resources are available to help you help your child are all useful.

It is important to check in with yourself frequently about how you are feeling as it is stressful when you are learning that your child may indeed have a lifelong disability or illness. It can shatter your hopes and dreams for what you wanted your child's life to be versus the reality. However, being present with your child no matter what they are going through are dealing with can be so powerful to their life's experience. Your being present and engaged can also bring them much joy and motivate you to try to facilitate giving that to them. Also, learn about support groups that are available so you can communicate with other parents who are doing dealing with similar experiences.

Finding friends and family members who can be on your team and even give you a break when needed can be helpful. Often time so many parents of disabled children feel very isolated and overwhelmed by their child's needs. The other area of advocacy is within the educational system. Some educational advocates specialize in helping parents advocate for resources in the educational system. Now with so many services being administered online, this may allow for more possibilities with even respect to global relationships where educational advocates may be able to help parents navigate systems in different countries.

Parents can feel helpless and hopeless when confronted with numerous challenges while trying to care for their disabled child. We must allow space for children and families with disabilities in every area. A person with a disability should not have to feel limited but instead should feel that they can thrive despite certain challenges. That is the mentality of abundance that we want to instill in children with disabilities. So as a parent you may have to not take no for an answer when there is something you feel your child needs and is not getting. Your child may also learn not to take no for an answer when someone tells them they cannot do or achieve a particular dream. For example, children with disabilities can participate in sports, musical events, and a variety of other activities. Advances in the technological space will hopefully allow for cutting edge interventions to assist in improving functional outcomes.

22. My kids and I recently saw a homeless man who was missing an eye. I am worried that my son is now traumatized by this as he got very scared. What can I do to comfort him?

As a parent, you may try to shield your children from suffering or things that may scare them. When children witness deviations from what is typical or injuries and other evidence of suffering it can be scary. They may not understand why someone looks like that or worry about or whether something similar could happen to them or their loved ones. It is developmentally appropriate for children to have questions about things they see. You can just use it as an opportunity to discuss that some people are born differently some people have injuries and we should look at them through the lens of compassion.

Throughout time people collectively have expressed aversion to what is different and people who have disabilities have often been shunned from society. Again, you can instead use this as an opportunity to promote inclusivity and role model what that looks like to your children. It can also be a bridge to discussing other values around building a generous mindset to help those who are less fortunate. Teaching children to withhold judgement, accept people as they can be a valuable learning experience for them, reduce fear around differences, and grow their empathy.

If you catch your child staring, you can explain that some of these individuals are so used to people staring at them that instead it may be nice just to approach them in a way that makes them comfortable. Individuals with disabilities often deal with people staring at them or avoiding them completely because they are uncomfortable. Acknowledging appropriate curiosity can occur while you discuss who to reach out to someone, so they do not feel isolated and lonely.

23. What is a good way to get my children interested in STEM subjects?

So many young people shy away from science and math because it feels overwhelming, and it feels like something they cannot figure out. Yes, there is a degree of aptitude and the ability to learn certain things and you must understand your child's special needs or if they have learning disorders. The educational system that they are in should be understanding as well. One way is to find mentor figures who can help encourage your child.

I was part of a program in high school called "Medical Explorers" for minority students to get us in interested the healthcare sciences. Every week they would have a different doctor from a different specialty come to talk to us about their profession and we were even able to shadow them. Although not every child has these opportunities, this kind of exposure even virtually can be powerful and encourage a child to not give up.

Sometimes if not often, learning is very much about perseverance. Nowadays there are so many online resources, such as Khan Academy where children can watch videos about different stem subjects to improve their learning and curiosity. It is also important for them to understand that the book knowledge may be different from the experience of going into a certain profession, and later these aspects can merge even though it may seem tedious.

I think one of the most important things in encouraging children to be interested in STEM subjects involves showing them you believe in them. They may struggle but the important thing is if they keep trying. Having a STEM background can be valuable with future job opportunities which ebb and flow in different fields. Sometimes there is free tutoring available. Finding out what your child is learning about can help you keep your brain active by revisiting subjects or learning new things yourself and can help motivate them as well.

If they feel like they do not understand the subject, consider other resources to help them. If the frustration gets too much it is fine for them to take a mental break and then come back to it to tackle a challenge again. Overcoming challenges in education can bring a lot of fulfillment and it can improve their self-esteem through learning mastery. One bad grade or difficult subject should not deter a child from STEM education. It can be profound to have people around your child who do not give up on them and who believe in them.

In the US, minority students often deal with biases from teachers telling them they cannot achieve certain things or succeed in certain subjects. As a parent, you may have to be the one who teaches your child to fight that negativity and encourage them despite any force around them that tells them they cannot do otherwise. Those who do not give up often prevail at the end. It is also important that young girls are recruited into STEM subjects to even the playing field on a professional level and for their empowerment.

Finding ways to get your daughter feeling encouraged and interested, whether it is through science projects, mentoring opportunities, or volunteering even can be a great source of motivation. With a STEM education, you can still pursue arts, music, acting, and so many other fields. Humans do not have to do only one thing and have a better quality of life when they incorporate what they love doing.

Having some diverse skill sets can you help you explore different professional opportunities later in life. I have been able to pursue a career in medicine supplemented with my love for literature through reading and listening to audio books. I continue to pursue my love for the arts, particularly dancing as I am a trained Indian classical dancer. I feel I have been able to tap into my creative outlet professionally through medical journalism on the side. I would love for all young girls to feel that they can become whatever they want to be and not let educational roadblocks or other obstacles prevent them from believing so.

24. I found out I am HIV positive. When is the right time to tell children about something like this and what do I say?

The good news is that now with advances in the medical sciences, an HIV (human immunodeficiency virus) diagnosis has treatment options available that can greatly prolong life expectancy. Unfortunately, access to medication and cutting-edge treatments is difficult for many individuals with HIV across the world. The first thing you can do is advocating for yourself in your treatment making sure you have access to treatment. Humanitarian organizations like Doctors Without Borders can bring medication and treatment to communities in need so it is important to know if resources like this are accessible. It is also important that you focus on compliance with your treatment and taking care of your health to minimize your viral load.

You must go through your own grieving process and confrontation with mortality when given this diagnosis, so having a therapist to help you with it can be useful. It is important also not to succumb to feelings of shame or guilt and understand that this could happen to anyone. If you were engaged in repeated high-risk behaviors that increase your risk such as IV drug use, you must get help if that is an ongoing issue so that you do not jeopardize your health in other ways and can be present for your children. It is a personal decision went to tell your children, and it also depends on their developmental age. A young child may not understand complicated concepts of potential life expectancy and other elements of time, which may lead them to worry you will die very soon. Appreciating confusion around this may allow you to reassure them that is a condition that needs treatment, and that you are taking measures to protect your health so you can be there for them. A skilled therapist can help you navigate difficult conversations with your child about your diagnosis, explaining what HIV is, what it means for the family.

If they noticed you were taking medicine you may introduce the topic by saying, "I have to take medicine for this condition (a type of sickness) to keep me healthy." You can allow them to ask questions. Also, you must keep in mind a bit about privacy. The diagnosis is your medical information no one needs to know about it and unfortunately, in society, there is still a stigma attached which makes people not want to share. If your child knows, please understand they may want talk about it at school with friends or teachers or other family members and family friends.

This is normal, and you do not necessarily want your child to grow up thinking this is some dirty secret they cannot be shared because that just is further stigmatizing and isolating for your child. It is understandable that you also do not want your child being shunned, stigmatized, made fun of, or avoided if they disclose this information. You can explain like some people might have certain things they have to take medicine for like high blood pressure so that they do not get sick. You can explain that perhaps you do not want to share this information with many people, with also understanding that a child's emotional process may come present in conversation with others, drawings, or through play. If privacy is paramount, you can share what you feel comfortable sharing with your child with the knowledge they may speak about it.

As your child gets older and they have a better understanding of the difference between a condition that you manage overtime versus something more acute, then you may want to talk about this in more detail. You may decide you do not want to scare your young child especially if you are otherwise healthy. For children thinking their parent is sick may make them fearful and you introduce them to the topic in a way that can manage this fear. As they get older into their teenage years, you can discuss with them what this means more long-term and the plan you have in place for managing any issues can come up with respect to your health.

You can also give them hope by saying that researchers are working on possible cures like vaccines and other treatments. Sometimes what you are dealing with can help to teach a child about protecting their health and being safe with their lifestyle choices. You can use it as an opportunity to explain that sometimes we make one minor lapse in judgment and it can have risks such as that which comes with unprotected sexual activity or intravenous drug use. It can serve as a valuable learning opportunity.

Some children see their parents struggling with illness because of a long-standing smoking habit and it can deter them from wanting to experience the same thing. I have a family history of diabetes and as much as I love sweets (and I was cursed with a sweet tooth), I do think about ways of mitigating my risk and try to moderate the number of sweets I consume in my diet. I will not say I do the best job of it consistently, but I am also a work in progress! I also try to focus on healthy lifestyle habits such as exercising to further mitigate my risk. So sometimes illnesses in the family can teach your children how to navigate their lives in a different way to maintain optimal health and that can ultimately be positive. It can also make them anxious about their health and getting sick as well, so that response should be monitored as well.

25. I do not want to get my 11-year-old daughter a cell phone. All her friends have them, so she feels like I am being unfair. I want her to be able to contact me in an emergency and of course would want to know about her whereabouts, but I do not feel she needs a cell phone right now. Is it smart to get her a phone of her own or should I stick to my resolve to say no to her?

Cell phones present a modern-day technology conundrum that parents were perhaps partly fortunate to avoid in previous generations. There are pros and cons with a child having access to a cell phone. Let us examine the pros. Devices with a GPS tracking system allow you to know your child's whereabouts if they do not willfully disable it. I have had teenage patients who left their phone at a friend's house so that their parents think that they are at a sleepover, while they wandered the streets at night, at times putting themselves at risk. However, even with that risk, the possibility of maintaining steady contact gives many parents peace of mind when their children are not in their presence. Cell phones have a feature that can set off an alarm in case of danger. Cell phone plans can also limit usage of incoming and outgoing calls as well as text messages for better supervision.

There are also a variety of cons that come with cellular phones and other digital devices. Cell phones and plans tend to be a financial commitment, and children can add games and applications, adding to the cost often unknowingly to the child and parent. Cellular phones can put a child at risk for cyber bullying and leave a wide-open window for lurking predators looking to take advantage of vulnerable young people. There is also the risk of children posting and texting inappropriate messages and pictures. Children, and even adults, do not always understand the ramifications, and sometimes embarrassing content becomes public.

We live in an era of public shaming, which can raise awareness about injustices, such as police brutality, but it can also be personally damaging and allow for misinterpretation of events when a small clip is viewed of an incident. A group of college fraternity brothers was filmed on a phone, singing racist chants on a bus. Their families moved and the young men changed their names, but the posted video haunted them for years. This can influence job prospects, relationships, etc. The truth is, once this content gets online, it may stay there.

If you are going to get your young child a cell phone, then you must teach her how to handle social media and how she must protect herself from people who do not have good intentions. You can help her do this by establishing ground rules. It is useful to limit screen time or the use it as a small reward for completed homework and chores. Children can become addicted to cell phone use because of the constant stimulation it provides. The best way to counteract this is by limiting use and being consistent about, despite the objections you will invariably receive.

As the adult in the house, you should monitor your child's presence and activity on social media. Communicate with them about how to use the phone responsibly. Set guidelines and remind them that having a cell phone is a privilege that can be taken away if it is misused. Make sure to establish times that must be cell phone free, such as family meals or at night, right before and during bedtime. Children should not be falling asleep with their phones or hiding them under their pillow. That also includes role modeling the same as an adult. With cell phones often parents are expected to be continuously available to their employers, and this may help you set boundaries as well.

Have a conversation with your children on the economic limits of their cell phone use and agree on how much you are willing to contribute to their use. As children grow and you feel ready to give them a bit more independence that may be a time to consider getting them cellular phone, mostly for safety reasons. As a society, we are missing out on a lot due to our addiction to our devices. Recent research shows that social media use can cause depression and anxiety in adolescents, even more so in girls.[35] This is something to be taken into consideration when you decide what to do with your pre-adolescent daughter.

PART THREE

ADOLESCENCE

12 TO 14 YEARS

1. My 12-year-old African American son will be entering puberty soon. I am afraid that I am going to have to have that talk with him about racial profiling by police and police brutality. How do I address this with him?

Unfortunately, this question is a blaring reality for African Americans in the US. African American men are more likely to be viewed as aggressive, more likely to be racially profiled, and more likely to receive harsher legal sentences compared to white offenders, and they are more likely to be shot by the police.[1][2][3][4] Too many cases of police brutality toward African Americans and other minorities result in death or permanent disability. One example is the 2014 killing of 17-year-old Laquan McDonald, a black teen shot 16 times by a white police officer. Research has shown that police are more likely to view African American boys, even as young as ten, as older and less innocent.[5] This puts them at risk for more police violence if accused of a crime. This is compounded during adolescence as that is the time many children want more autonomy and independence, venturing out in the world more without their parents next to them.

Others killed by police include Tamir Rice, Botham Shem Jean, E.J. Bradford, George Floyd, Jamee Johnson, Antwon Rose, Stephon Clark, and Breonna Taylor.

An important part of talking to children about this difficult topic and how to interact with the police involves understanding their developmental stage. Younger children may not understand concepts such as racism and injustice, but a pre-pubescent or adolescent may understand these things better. For younger children, you may want to start by discussing historical examples of racial injustice and teach them about those who stood up for civil rights. That can assist with helping them understand that certain people over time were oppressed and treated inhumanely. You can explain to them how this has permeated across generations and still is an issue in the current day. It is important while discussing this somber topic, to still instill hope and optimism for the future. Dr. Martin Luther King role modeled that for us in many of his speeches. He did not shy away from talking about racial injustice and the deprivation of civil rights for people of color, but he spoke in a way that gave people hope that the future could be different. This is important as it allows a child feel agency instead of becoming hopeless about circumstances out of their control.

You can teach a child about civil rights by playing videos of Dr. King's speeches and discussing how he led a nonviolent movement. Other civil rights leaders such as Nelson Mandela have inspiring stories and books written about how they dealt with oppression and challenging it. It is useful for parents to familiarize themselves with some these books as we must protect future generations from similar situations. You can link how sometimes biases affect the way police respond to minorities.

You can tell your child that you want them to be safe and know how to handle themselves when they are confronted with the situation by a police officer. I tell my patients when they are confronted by a police officer to answer respectfully and cordially (which is so subjective when confounded with elements of bias of how speech is perceived based on preconceived ideas based on one's race). That does not mean things will necessarily be safe, but it can help. Yes, unfortunately, it is ridiculously unfair that the burden becomes on the African American child to do that, and it is good to explain how unfair that is. You can explain to them that sometimes police interactions do not go as they should.

I also tell my patients that they can answer their names but if other questions are asked, they can respond that they would like to call their parents or have a lawyer there before answering anything else. It is not up to a child to determine whether questions are safe are not. Interviews with African American police officers revealed that they recommend that even if a child has done something wrong, that they try to remain calm and compliant when interacting with the police.

Teenagers if they are driving should turn off the ignition and rolled down the window when the officer approaches. They should tell the officer before reaching for their license or registration that they are about to do so. Every officer has a badge number, and every police car has a license plate. It is good to encourage teenagers to remember these numbers especially if they are feeling violated in any way. Will these techniques guarantee against police brutality? There is no absolute guarantee but having a teenager who is informed about different possibilities when dealing with police interactions may help protect them.

2. I am worried my daughter is having unprotected sexual activity from some text messages I saw on her phone. How can I protect her?

It is natural for children to be curious about their bodies and as they grow older. They are under the influence of hormones which affect their feelings of attraction and curiosity about sexual activity. This is a normal part of development. The problem is sometimes we have the biological ability to do things that we are not exactly emotionally prepared for. Adolescence is also a period where there can be more impulsivity which can lead to them engaging in risky behaviors as a result.

The dangers of sexual activity at a young age include increased risk of sexually transmitted diseases, unwanted pregnancies which are also high-risk pregnancies at a young age, and the lack of emotional maturity. It can also set up a child to be victimized and mistreated. Navigating boundaries around sexual activity can be hard and without an external presence like a parent, and child may not be able to or feel disempowered to stop advances. You can have honest and open discussions with her about this, or have an outside party talk to her about this. Supervision allows for you to monitor her behavior so that she does not put herself at risk.

Adolescents also want to be around friends and socialize as this is the natural part of development. It is important to allow for that social development, but you can do it in a supervised fashion. Having your daughter allow friends to come over for healthy interaction can help you supervise a little better. There is a fine balance between stifling your teen and allowing them to have some autonomy which is a natural drive as young people grow older. Regardless your daughter should be aware of the risks of sexual activity at a younger age without being shamed and she should be educated about how to keep herself safe.

3. My 12-year-old daughter attends a rigorous school, but she recently started having panic attacks before quizzes or tests. Is this a sign she is under a lot of pressure and is there something I should do about it? If she does not keep up her grades, she could lose her spot in the school and that might ruin her chances of going to a good high school and then a top-notch university.

Test-taking anxiety may reflect feeling overwhelmed and stress. Stress can be positive if it challenges and motivates someone, so some anxiety can be beneficial to achieving goals. The problem is when it is overwhelming, it causes physical health problems such as stomach aches and panic attacks and impacts functioning. You do not want children to go through their adolescence not being able to enjoy themselves for the same. Learning and achieving goals is also a journey, and you want it to be a positive experience. I meet a lot of parents who knowingly or unknowingly want to live vicariously through their children. They have high expectations because they were high achieving or because they know their children have opportunities that they did not and do not want them to squander them.

Parents often worry about their children's future job placement and security, having the proper educational credentials to get good positions. They also worry that their child will not have self-esteem, be able to care for themselves, and make better decisions for themselves. Often there is often undue importance placed on which university of child attends, and some parents become hyper-focused on getting their child into a premier institution. There is also a fierce competition that impacts the pressure students feel. Many students can get a great education at less cost depending on available resources.

Malcolm Gladwell describes in his book "David and Goliath," that students may drop out of STEM careers when they become demoralized being in an extremely competitive school, but they may continue to get advanced degrees if they were in a less competitive school. Understandably, you may want your child to actualize the potential you see in them. It is also important to understand that as a parent you cannot be completely objective. This means that you may be pushing them harder than they can tolerate or in such a way that is not considered healthy motivation. It can also backfire in the form of them being rebellious or becoming stressed out. I find that this shift in perspective can be hard for parents where they take a position of letting go a little bit and allowing the child to work at their own pace.

You could encourage your child by telling them that it is the effort that matters and if they are learning and trying, that is the most important thing. Taking away all enjoyment for an entire summer because they do not get perfect grades may not be productive in the long run. You also remind yourself that your children are not alive to live your dreams they must find their own way. You can have certain expectations, but it is important not to jeopardize their mental health in the process.

Parents may think, so then should I not pressure them at all, and should I have no expectations? Should I just let them do whatever they want like be on their electronic device all day without doing their schoolwork? No, it does not mean letting go of parenting or appropriate discipline. Parents that do not enforce any discipline and act more like friends to their children can be detrimental to a child's wellbeing. They may not impose necessary boundaries with their parenting, which then facilitates an environment where their children can make impulsive decisions with limited judgment.

Therefore, you want to strike a balance where you are encouraging and motivating to your child by letting them know you believe in them. You do not want them to be so nervous and so stressed that they cannot perform. I know of students who throw up before a test because they become so anxious. This is not healthy, and these are not the coping mechanisms you want your child to develop to deal with stress. Performance anxiety can happen even without external pressure, however. Therapy can help manage it and sometimes if it inhibits functioning enough, medication management maybe helpful. This is to be discussed with your child's doctor.

4. I overheard my 13-year-old son speaking to his friends in a derogatory manner about girls. I want my son to respect girls and women. How do I address this with him?

Role modeling ways to address sexism and misogyny is important because in essence it is a form of oppressive bullying and is harmful. Women have lost lives because of misogyny and sexism. When you hear this, it may be useful to talk to your son about this in private afterward. Or if you can without humiliating him, you can discuss it in front of the group as a teaching lesson. We should learn to speak about women respectfully. Men and women should be able to show mutual respect. Teach your son about concepts against objectifying women and degrading them. The more this is done even in smaller interactions, it can cultivate a general appreciation for women and respect.

If you do not address it, sometimes these behaviors can continue and escalate. You can share with your son stories of historical and current events where women have not been treated well at all. Women have been burned or stoned for being a woman, have been labeled as witches, have been denied voting rights, equal pay, and suffered a variety of sexual harassment assaults throughout of their lifetime. Young boys may not be at an age ready to process some of the more brutal aspects of sexism, but you can continue to educate young children about fairness and equality in a developmentally appropriate way.

How do you talk about other women in the household? How did the men in your family treat other women? How did they talk about women? You want to expose your child to people who respect and value strong women and the more you do that hopefully the more they learn to do the same. It is not always easy if you are in a home with another man or men who are misogynistic. Often women may also speak poorly of other women representing internalized sexism projected by demeaning another.

Understanding yourself and the world around you concerning how women are treated is important to help your son learn to be different. Instead of chastisement or harassment of your son, you could simply say why do you feel the need to talk about a girl this way? How does it make you feel? Is that the way you would want your sister or mother to be spoken about? Is it the right thing to do? Facilitating this type of inquiry in an open honest way without anger may help your son think about it and reflect on it. It may also help his friends do the same. His friends may be in homes where misogyny and sexism are so rampant that they do not know any differently and do not question it. Much of the world lives in a patriarchal society where women are not spoken about or dealt with respectfully manner. We must change this, and it starts with smaller actions like preventing the formation of sexist beliefs in our children.

We must show support, and fight forms of oppression both systematically and interpersonally. Let us all reject negative portrayals of women in the media; remember that advertisers are in the business to sell, not empower. Let us hold each other accountable so that we do not use gender-laden terms that demean women. Let us find ways to mentor, encourage, and build the self-esteem of girls and women, whether it is through our jobs or within our family and friend circles.

5. My 13-year-old daughter has been more withdrawn recently. We moved to the suburbs from the city this year and she started a new school, which is ethnically less diverse. She is Indian and now her classmates are mostly Caucasian. Now we notice that after dinner she usually just isolates herself in her room and does not want to socialize much with the family. She does not talk to us much at all about her day. We are a close family, so this is concerning. Her grades have dropped a bit, too, but we think it is because of transitioning to a different school. How do we get her to be more open with us?

Moving schools can be stressful. Sometimes, it means adjusting to a different course curriculum. It always involves meeting new peers and making new friends, which means navigating all of that and trying to fit in as easily as possible. For a minority child, moving to a different ethnic environment may be startling. This can be true for children who move from rural environments to more urban communities, children attending school with those of different socioeconomic backgrounds, etc. Other children may not understand how to interact with someone "different" because whether they realize it or not, they may have developed stereotypes and stigmas, which they have picked up from their elders or neighbors. When my family moved from the inner city of Pittsburgh to the suburbs it was a similar situation. I was asked by a teacher one day about what would happen if I got married and my husband happened to die before me. He told me he heard Indian women jump into a fire after the loss of a husband and asked if I would do the same. This was a question asked out of genuine curiosity, but It was startling to me as a teenager who wanted to be treated like everyone else.

Micro and macroaggressions can be more painful and hurtful. Research shows that racism affects children, without a doubt. It can cause depression and symptoms of anxiety.[6] It would be helpful if your daughter had someone she could trust to talk to about her experience, such as a therapist who understands cross-cultural experiences. As a child psychiatrist who is a member of a minority population myself, I see many people who consider themselves culturally informed and sensitive, but they do not have any specific training or experience that allows them to be genuinely effective. This translates into a lot of their patients not feeling understood.

I once had a supervisor who did not understand some of the sacrifices my parents made and how many immigrants must deal with the challenge of separating from their families to provide their children a better life. This is often lost on a person who has not experienced any of this and views it more as a choice that was made. It would be reasonable to ask your daughter if she is being treated well by other students and teachers. You should ask if she feels bullied or even just misunderstood for having some differences from her peers. It would be useful to find out if she feels pressure to perform academically, and that if it is a struggle for her to keep up. Many immigrant families emphasize academic achievement, leaving children to often feel a lot of pressure to perform.

Try to find out what environmental stresses she is experiencing. As a child psychiatrist, I would order some lab work to determine any medical issues could be affecting her. For example, a child may be anemic or have thyroid that is under-functioning. Once any medical issue is ruled out, it would be appropriate for this adolescent girl to be evaluated for depressive symptoms. She could be isolating herself because she feels misunderstood or because she is suffering from some depressive symptoms. This could also be a time-limited phenomenon, such as that seen with what is known as an adjustment disorder. If that is the case, it is important to get her to a safe place emotionally where she feels she has someone she can speak to while receiving the gentle encouragement she needs.

6. My 14-year-old daughter asked me why men in power seem often get away with sexually harassing women. How do I answer this?

When people in leadership positions have allegations of sexual harassment or assault, it may seem like justice has not been served and people can get away with this kind of behavior. The reality is that men of power often do get away with sexual harassment. Even when litigation takes place, many will settle out of court and the victims must sign nondisclosure agreements, so it does not become public information. There is often a lot of victim-blaming as well and public shaming of the victims, often being accused of trying to extort money by making false allegations.

This does not just happen in the context of politics, but pretty much in every profession, there have been instances of sexual harassment towards women. Women who have been victimized are more likely to be re-victimized, which continues to cycle.[7] Although this is the case, you must teach your daughter not to become disempowered. She should still stand up for herself and become capable of exiting an uncomfortable situation if possible. She must feel comfortable approaching a trusted adult if she is victimized or even if she has questions about someone's behavior.

Men in leadership positions can take advantage of their power by seducing their subordinates. There are also many instances where justice has been served. The *Me Too* movement has permeated worldwide where women are standing up for each other and women's rights. Allowing your daughter to get a self-defense lesson can help her learn how to defend herself which may also save her life one day. In certain parts of the world where there is a lot of violence towards women, a woman sometimes has few choices and risks losing her life if she tries to defend herself. This highlights why it is important to be aware of and contribute to causes that help empower women worldwide.

Allowing your daughter to see the work of various organizations that are focused on female empowerment may encourage her to get involved. It is important that young people feel there are adults out there who will keep them safe and protect them. It is also important that they see justice being served appropriately. This of course varies depending on local governments. The key is educating your daughter that even if it looks like a lot of people get away with things like this, it is not acceptable behavior.

7. My son came home with a skull tattoo. He is 14 and I am mortified. How do I handle this?

In the US, the legal age to get a tattoo is 18. This helps prevent younger adolescents from making impulsive decisions that they may later regret like tattoos. Tattoos can be a source of regret even when one chooses to get them in adulthood. First, the most important thing is to find out if it was done with a sterile needle and to make sure your son is up to date on vaccinations such as hepatitis B and tetanus. It would not be a bad idea to speak to a doctor about this. Secondly, you want to make sure there is no infection developing on the tattoo site.

A healing tattoo should be treated like a wound and keeping the area clean and with a dressing if needed especially if it is rubbing against clothing. It is understandable to be upset about your child having permanent ink applied body.

It can also be very frustrating that your son did not abide by rules that were established such as not getting tattoos. One consolation is that nowadays tattoos do not have to be permanent. There exists the laser tattoo removal process available which over repeated sessions can cause a tattoo to be removed. Of course, this is much harder when it is a large tattoo, and it can be expensive, but it is a technology that works well. There are complications of tattoos such as reactions to the ink, possibility of infection, etc. Also, there is a possibility of blood-borne diseases if the needle is not sterile. You can talk to your son about how sometimes tattoos can influence other people's perceptions. This sometimes is something that can be noticed by potential employers, especially if you are in a job working with young people who may be influenced into getting a tattoo because they see a trusted adult with one.

Often the decision to get a tattoo is not made in young people thinking about our potential future ramifications. You may not have any control when your son becomes an adult over the tattoos that he gets. In some cultures, a tattoo is culturally sanctioned and is a common thing to do. In some cultures, a tattoo can have religious significance. Sometimes I have had patients who instead of cutting themselves they switch to other forms of causing injury to the body such as multiple piercings, tattoos, etc. Often the idea of getting a tattoo has to do with the novelty of it and for a lot of people, once they get it, they may realize they do not even like it that much. I educate my patients about the trend of earlobe expanders and how that can eventually cause their earlobes to even rip, requiring surgery to fix it. Once they have this information, it is up to them to decide what to do with it. Likewise, you can have an honest discussion with your teenage son about your concerns over this.

8. My 14-year-old daughter's classmate recently died by suicide. How do I talk to her about this, and will it make her more at risk for the same thing?

According to the Centers for Disease Control and Prevention (CDC) WISQARS Leading Causes of Death Reports in 2018, suicide is the second leading cause of death in individuals ages 10-34. You can take the approach of gently ask her how she is feeling about what happened to her classmate. For young people even if they are not close to the person who died, if they were classmates or peers, it can still affect them profoundly. If you can find out what the school is doing about this such as whether they have talked to the students about what happened, and do they have any grief counseling available? Sometimes it is helpful for young people to participate in a memorial or a small way of recognizing the person who passed whether it is through writing a letter or otherwise.

You can allow your daughter to talk as she feels comfortable without pushing her too hard. It is reasonable to ask her how she has been feeling in general and whether she has ever had these thoughts. You can tell her that if she ever feels down or hopeless, that she can come to talk to you or another trusted adult or a therapist. Suicide always has a big ripple effect that can touch a lot of people in different ways. There have been reports of contagion effect resulting in increased suicidal ideation and behavior after exposure to suicide within school districts.[8]

In general, it is not a bad idea to make sure there is no access to means. Unlocked firearms, pill bottles that are accessible, and cleaning substances can be used to engage in suicidal behavior. If it seems like your child is dealing with some symptoms of depression, it is even more important to assess accessibility to lethal means. Firearms should be locked and unloaded. This may also be an opportunity to talk with other parents about how you all can support your children and help mitigate stress.

It can be hard to identify when a child needs help. Sometimes if not often, young people do not feel comfortable talking to their parents about how they are feeling so having an outsider involved can be helpful. You also want to check your responses to this event. Constantly worrying that your child may do the same because it happens in the school may increase your anxiety and ability to be present with your child. Being mindful that mental health should be a priority when considering your child's overall well-being.

A lot of parents avoid those who lost someone by suicide and those families tend to feel isolated. It can also be an act of compassion to reach out to those parents and think about what you can do for those families. This may be in the form of dropping off some food, sharing books or other resources or just being there for them. Losing a child by suicide can be a very lonely experience for parents. It can be hard to engage them when you cherish your children's milestones and feel hesitant to share that with them out of guilt of hurting them, so you may just avoid them instead. People also do not realize that it maybe triggering for the parent who has lost a child to be expected to celebrate another child's milestones. The best thing is to be there for them empathically and be mindful that their pain is monumental, to be considerate of that when you celebrate children's milestones, but to also involve them in a way that feels supportive.

It is important to have empathy, sensitivity to their loss, and understand the pain involved in seeing other families move on and their children growing up. Anyone who suffered a great loss can take it out on those around them by being short or snapping at others. If you have difficulty with how they are treating you, you can show your love from a distance, gently reminding them you are there but giving them some space. People do remember those who reach out. Remembering the birthday of the child who passed and reaching out can be very meaningful to the parents. Checking in on them from time to time is a nice and sometimes welcome gesture of support. Assuming that things are not okay after such a loss and never will be the same can help you develop compassion for their journey.

9. My 14-year-old son wants to play tackle (American) football. I am worried about his brain being injured. Is it all right for me to forbid this or will he resent me?

There is growing definitive research about the dangers of tackle football concerning concussions and traumatic brain injury. Repeated concussions can cause injury to the developing brain.[9] Some schools have implemented more stringent protocols to protect children. However, the enforcement of this is variable. A lot of people look back fondly at their days on a sports team and feel that it kept them out of trouble. Tackling, unfortunately, makes one more prone to various injurious including brain injuries. If you can find another sport for your son to be engaged in that puts him at less risk, that could mitigate brain related injury. There are many adults who felt that participating in the sport in high school allowed them to learn teamwork, helped them to focus on academics, and they were able to stay safe without much injury. It can be helpful to discuss safety protocols and your concerns with coaches and your son's doctor.

10. I am the father of two teenage girls, ages 13 and 15. Their mother and I were young when we had them. We both had to work blue-collar jobs to support the family and could not focus on higher educational pursuits we may have enjoyed if we had not had kids so young. How do I teach my daughters to become strong girls and women?

One day, when my niece was four years old, I gave her some almond milk. She drank it down with great confidence. "My mommy says if I drink milk, I'm going to grow up to be big and strong," she said to me and her brother. Later that day, as I sat in my office, I reflected on what happens to girls that age a decade later in their life.

Many of them come to see me, feeling insecure about the way they look and how others view them. In some minority communities, girls are often taught to be embarrassed about having a darker complexion. Some develop eating disorders to physically diminish the amount of space they take up, and many do not feel accepted for who they are.

Research shows that young children have high self-esteem, but it decreases during adolescence, particularly in girls. This gender gap continues into adulthood.[10][11][12] The media is relentless in the images and messages it puts out that the worth of a woman depends on her physical attractiveness. Women with successful, busy careers are often portrayed as less than fun and described as "aggressive" instead of assertive. Research supports the concept that men are willing to compete for professional opportunities more than women.[13][14]

This belief system sometimes guides a woman to shy away from certain career choices, which limit her chances for advancement. As all this continues to unfold, fathers concentrate on protecting their young daughters from things like sexual harassment. Instead of focusing on the salacious details of specific acts, it would be useful to look at harassment as part of a continuum. When we look at an act of harassment, we must consider what happens before and after. First, someone feels the need to belittle a woman, to make her feel less than, and then take advantage of her. The psychological insult that ensues in the aftermath of the actual harassment makes a woman vulnerable to it happen again. Far too often, the cycle repeats.

We know that women are paid less than men for doing the same amount of work.[15] Women are given the message that professional and personal successes are binary, that you cannot have both, so you better choose. Research shows that women who work, as opposed to only doing household chores, have longer days, without any reduction in their domestic responsibilities.[16] All over the world, even when women have illustrative careers, they can still be marginalized and oppressed socially, by society in general, or by families they marry into. These are all reasons why the empowerment of young girls and women is so vital in reducing issues like harassment.

When women are empowered, they are less vulnerable, less likely to be victimized, and less likely to be re-victimized. Companies with organizational policies to address harassment in the workplace foster a culture that empowers women. This reduces symptoms of post-traumatic stress disorder in women who have experienced intimate partner violence. As a psychiatrist, I think we must learn and teach these basic principles. Girls and women are individuals innately worthy of love, regardless of their appearance, accomplishments, or ability to cook. We do not have to take advice that feels intuitively wrong or harmful.

We must never judge women who stay in domestic violence situations, as studies show that women sometimes be at a higher risk of being killed when they try to flee.[17] It is more helpful to show support and assist them in allocating resources. I encourage girls and women to study profiles and tactics of women leaders who have successfully overcome hurdles, such as harassment, and gone on to live integrated lives. I tell them to surround themselves with people who believe in them and offer support, and encouragement. A woman can focus on her own personal growth by avoiding or minimizing interaction with those who drain energy, seeking and creating opportunities, such as mentoring and training, which provide avenues to advance professional skills and improve versatility. For a woman facing harassment, talking to someone like a trusted supervisor at work, a colleague who will listen and believe her can be a source of support. If the harassment happens at the workplace, finding out what policies exist to protect employees can help her understanding of what avenues to take to address this.

Exposing young girls to STEM careers can increase interest and motivation. Encourage your daughters to read books and watch documentaries about inspiring women who have overcome challenges to become educated and contribute to society in a meaningful way. Find mentorship programs that may be available to help guide your daughters with furthering their education or possible career choices. Far too many women are sold the idea that they must choose between a career and a family, that it is not possible to have both. Nobody tells men this, so why do women have to make a binary choice?

I have many female colleagues who lacked the appropriate mentorship when it came to their career. Some became burned out from working hard without any chance of promotion, so they discontinued their career path. They lacked perseverance because they did not have adequate support. I have seen male colleagues figure out how to advance their careers while spending meaningful time with their families. Why can't women being supported to do the same thing? In life people make difficult choices, sometimes it is about taking care of loved ones and having to sacrifice professional aspirations to do that. There should be equality between the sexes for these life responsibilities as well.

Girls need to be taught to speak up for themselves and demand more, to be treated as equals deserving of a seat at the table. This is a systematic issue because oppressive environments prevent girls from speaking up. This conditioning should begin at a young age, so they build these skills. I meet many girls with a family background like this father and his daughters. I encourage them to read and give difficult subjects a try because they can achieve great things. When I asked my little niece what she wants to be when she gets older, she said, "an artist, a doctor, and a teacher!" I loved that she did not even try to limit herself to one domain. Pursuing our creative interests can enrich our lives in so many ways and provide an outlet to the monotony and routine of other jobs. Fashion entrepreneur Stacey Bendet says, "Here's to strong women. May we know them, may we be them, and may we raise them!"

11. My son does not know that his stepdad is not his biological father. Is it wrong to keep the truth from him? Should I just tell him?

Now with various DNA testing kits, it is becoming more common that people are finding out more details about their biological roots. Finding out this information at a later age can make a child feel betrayed and result in complicated feelings. It is better to be transparent with children from a young age. I have had a patient who did not know her father was her stepfather, but it was clear that her biological father was a different race than her mom as the child was bi-racial. This caused confusion for the child regarding not being able to understand her origins.

If needed, entrust the help of a therapist on how best to do this. Your child may have a lot of questions, particularly about his birth father and express curiosity. This is normal and expected. It is important not to put down the birth father with derogatory language when discussing this with your son. Some children find out their birth fathers are incarcerated or are a donor. They may express a desire to meet them or fear expressing that desire to their mother and stepparent worrying they will disappoint them. If they do not bring it up, it does not mean they do not think about it, and that it will not come up more as an unfinished chapter in their life later.

Many parents and stepparents in this situation may feel insecure if their child wants to reach out their birth father. Mothers may think that it is a bad idea for the child to communicate, especially if the birth father demonstrated abusive behavior towards the mother and they believe it would be harmful to the child. There can be monitored visits with a social worker or another trusted third party and the birth father which may help keep boundaries if there are those concerns. This is often decided by a judge or Child Protective Services.

It is natural for the child to still be curious and want to know more. It may be too much to process for a young child to find out if their father is incarcerated for a charge such as murder, so you may want to delay that detail until they are older. However, allowing your child to express their feelings is a good thing and allows them to process this information with loving support. The issue of a child being born via a donor can be challenging to know how to navigate this, a child may want to meet the donor now or at a later age. The donor may be open to communication or they may not be, which can cause feelings of betrayal. You can talk to a professional who is intimately aware of these circumstances and the psychological issues that come up for children and get more insight on how to assist your child through this.

12. My husband's friends like to smoke marijuana at parties. I do not want my children to see this. He still wants to go to these "family parties," according to his friends. Am I being too rigid?

The reality is that when children are running around parties they do see, smell, and inhale things that are going around going on around them. There are some logistical questions like is this done after the children are asleep at night and there are responsible adults who are not under the influence? Is it done inside or outdoors because if it is done inside, and are now exposing your child to secondhand smoke and the smell of marijuana? Marijuana has deleterious effects on the developing brain, so you do not want your child to have exposure.[18]

This can be hard when there is a disagreement between you and your spouse and the social circle you are part of. Ultimately you should do what you think is a responsible decision for your children. If you do not want them to be exposed and this is going to be an ongoing issue, then you may have to refrain from attending or having your children attend. Your husband may decide to take the children himself which can also be an issue. Explaining to him how you do not want children to grow up and engaging behaviors that can be harmful to them may be useful.

Some adults smoke cigars at parties as part of a ritual that they enjoy. If it is occasional use in this fashion that you can mostly shield your children from secondhand smoke, and if it is done outdoors away from children occasionally, it may be tolerable for you. The issue becomes one it is part of a lifestyle that is regular and avoiding it becomes impossible. If that is the case it may be useful to get support from an outside organization like Al-Anon or an outside therapist to help you deal with this. You are right to be concerned about this and it does not mean that you are just being prudish.

13. Our 13-year-old daughter seems to be obsessed with exercising. She has been spending three hours a day exercising. Does she have a disorder?

It would be good to find out what your daughter's views are about her own body image in an empathic manner. Does she feel like she needs to lose weight and is that the purpose for exercising? With respect to exercise in general, it is not natural for children to sit in a classroom for eight hours a day without a lot of physical activity. In fact, there should be a balance between how much a child studies versus physical activity, so it is healthy for children to engage in exercise. With that said when it is excessive or related to an eating disorder that can grow to be a bigger problem.

Children who are engaged in sports like ballet may feel pressure by the cultural environment to stay thin. Sometimes children feel this way after being bullied at school about how they look. Sometimes children enjoy the type of exercise they are doing. For example, I learned Indian classical dance growing up. I loved it so much that I would often practice by myself every day because I enjoyed it. If your daughter is doing high-intensity workout for three hours straight like running on a treadmill that can cause injury to the body, and if it is for the purpose of weight loss, it is a form of restrictive behavior. This is different from engaging in an activity that can be time-consuming but is enjoyable.

I have a friend who has two daughters that love participating in gymnastics and they spend a good portion of the week going to practices and meets. They were able to maintain their grades at school and function well overall socially, without being enticed into bad habits. Being involved in regular physical activity or sport can really help children build pro-social skills, challenge their brain in different ways, and help them learn the art of teamwork. If your daughter seems to be overdoing it to you, get the help of the therapist. Exercise is a great way to relieve stress and reduce anxiety as well as elevate mood if done in a healthy way that is not excessive. People with eating disorders often have waxing and waning symptoms a different part of their lives. They constantly try to diet, take up different extreme sports, or engage in excessive exercise to lose weight, and sometimes it can get so severe that it physically threatens their life. When symptoms are so severe and the weight loss is profound, they may require inpatient treatment at an eating disorder program for stabilization with long term maintenance treatment.

14. How can I supervise my kids on social media?

Social media can be positive in respect to finding people who share your hobbies and interests, forming friendships, staying in touch with people. There are even opportunities for learning new things and being aware of current events. However, there is research showing that it is associated with depression and anxiety during adolescence.[19] Also, social media allows for predatory behavior, cyberstalking, and cyberbullying, as well as other dangers. It can be hard to keep up to date with all the advances in technology as young people also learn tricks about how to get access to sites and platforms that adults are not aware of.

There are parental safeguard controls that you can utilize, and you can also have them only use it around you, which gets harder to control as a child ages as they demand more independence. Sometimes young people post things that they later regret as well so you can monitor that activity. The best way to supervise the use of digital technology is to set limits. For example, allowing your child to be with their device late at night when they should be sleeping creates more opportunities for them to be affected by negative effects of social media use.

Social media also creates an atmosphere where comparisons to others can make people feel bad about themselves. Viewing carefully curated photo shopped images of people may increase insecurity. When I was younger, I wanted a subscription to Seventeen magazine and my father gently refused, saying he did not think that was a good idea. He did not want me to be exposed to certain messaging and beauty standards that would affect my self-esteem.

With the pandemic, it has become harder to control technology use because children must use it for schoolwork. However, I do know many parents who have been good about making sure the device is removed from the child's hands well before bedtime, giving them adequate time to wind down at night before falling asleep. One discussion to have before allowing your child access is to establish the rules. A child should know that having the privilege of owning a digital device also means that there will be limits set on use.

You should know the social media sites your child is using and monitor the content. It is important is having a discussion with your child about the dangers of social media use and encouraging them to make decisions using good judgment. Learning how to not take things personally may also be a useful skillset to develop while engaging in social media use. That does not mean your child should be subjected to various forms of cyberbullying, but if they run across something unkind about them you can teach them how to manage their emotions and not let their self-esteem be affected.

15. My 14-year-old son has panic attacks before tests in high school. During these attacks, he sweats, says his heart races, and he feels like he is going to die. How do I help him overcome this test anxiety?

Anxiety is common among children. Sometimes it is situational, triggered by speaking in front of people or taking tests. The good news is, there are effective techniques exist to deal with anxiety. For example, research shows that mindfulness techniques can help reduce anxiety among young people.[20] When stress severely impacts a child's functioning, certain integrative treatments and medications can help. That is a conversation to have with a pediatrician or child psychiatrist.

Scientists have found that the brain is organized by an extrinsic and intrinsic network. The extrinsic network becomes activated when we do tasks, such as preparing a meal or getting dressed.

The intrinsic network becomes activated when we engage in self-reflection and focus on our emotions.[21][22][23][24][25][26][27] These two networks are rarely active at the same time, which allows us to focus on tasks without being distracted.[28][29][30][31]

Research by Dr. Zoran Josipovic at New York University has used neuroimaging studies on the brains of Buddhist monks and experienced mediators and shows that these individuals can activate both networks at the same time.[32][33] According to Dr. Josipovic, this may prove to be neuroprotective while providing a better sense of personal harmony. Imagine if your child (and you) could approach your emotional reactions in a more objective manner, such as completing tasks that do not require much thought, like washing dishes. You could approach emotional triggers and disappointments from a place of serenity and peace. An employer or a leader who can regulate their emotions and communicate effectively can have a more collaborative, productive relationship with those they supervise.

The Tibetan people have a spiritual and secular leader known as the Dalai Lama. This anointment dates back 600 years. Tenzin Gyatso was deemed the 14th Dalai Lama in 1937, at age two. He was forced to flee Tibet into exile in 1959 and has been living in the village of Dharamsala in Northern India. A serious meditator, the Dalai Lama reports turning in at nine p.m. and waking up around three a.m. to begin his five hours of daily meditation. He uses different kinds of techniques during his practice, such as single point meditation in which you concentrate on one entity or object. There are mindfulness meditation exercises you can practice with your child to help him manage his anxiety. You can practice this yourself and guide your child to do it, too, with you or by himself. Encourage focusing on the breath while observing the air going in and out of your body. Here are some tips on meditating:

An Exercise in Mindfulness

Wear comfortable relaxed clothing, find a quiet room, and sit. Light a candle and dim the lights if that helps you to relax. Picture something you feel connected to, such as the ocean or a God you believe in. Sit with your legs folded and back straight, or in a chair with both feet on the ground. Close your eyes. Imagine yourself somewhere peaceful, like the beach, or simply think of nothing at all. Take deep, slow breaths in and out. Thoughts will infiltrate your mind but try not to get frustrated when that happens. Gently remove them and try to retain focus. Say or think the word "Om," pronounced long and slow like "Aum." Repeat slowly. If you feel frustrated by thoughts entering your mind, do not worry. Meditation takes practice.

Even monks who practice hours of meditation a day become frustrated at times. Imagine a broom, gently sweeping away the thoughts entering your mind. When you feel more comfortable, focus your attention on your breath. Observe your breath coming in and out of your body, slow the rate of your breathing down so that you take deep and slow breaths.

Over time, you can incorporate other types of meditation, such as analytical meditation. This involves utilizing a more cognitive behavioral technique, which is a mental health practice. You focus on examining a problem that you have or a difficult interaction you had with someone. Try to develop empathy for the other party and seek to understand your feelings. Begin by practicing mindfulness for five minutes, then increase the time as tolerated. Journaling any changes, you have noticed after a few weeks of this practice can help you reflect on potential differences in irritability, frustration tolerance. Try to incorporate daily exercise and meditation into your routine.

There are many parallels between analytical meditation and

cognitive-behavioral therapy, which utilize mental health treatments. Cognitive-behavioral therapy involves analyzing a situation by breaking it down into your thoughts and feelings.[34] [35] You then think of alternative thoughts, which can result in alternative feelings that are more positive. In cognitive behavioral therapy, you do repetitive exercises to train your mind to implement these techniques automatically.[36]

One such exercise involves writing about a situation that caused the negative feeling, like being angry or upset. You list the thoughts that you had about that situation and how it made you feel. For example, let us say you were upset earlier in the day because someone in another car cut you off abruptly while you were driving. You may have felt angry. That feeling has a pre-existing thought attached to it. Feelings arise from thoughts. You may have thought to yourself, "I can't believe this person just did this," or "this person just disrespected me," or "this person has no concern for other people's safety and could have caused a bad car accident." This may make you feel angry, upset, and even vengeful.

When confronted with these emotions, try to think alternative thoughts. What if this person was rushing to an emergency room for a medical emergency? What if this person just found out that a loved one has passed away? What if she or had a difficult interpersonal interaction earlier in the day? Mindfulness can help when you are flooded with emotions by slowing down the thought process and preventing hasty reactions. The same is true for your child. A therapist can work on changing the internal language so there is a different response to calm and center any automatic negative thoughts while also reducing anxiety.

16. I worry my 16-year-old daughter sees celebrities like Kyle Jenner and thinks that is realistic for her future, not to go to college and have a billion-dollar business. How do I explain that this is unlikely for most people?

There is a duality that comes with celebrities. On the one hand, their persona sometimes allows for the imaginative process where a child can dream big to achieve certain things. On the other hand, it can set up a pretense of unrealistic expectations. The confounding factor here is that we also live in a world where young people are making money for being social media influencers with YouTube channels etc.

When young people believe that if they pursue a certain subjective image, it will guarantee success, that can be set up for lots of disappointment. The reality is that most young mothers of Kylie Jenner's age do not have the financial freedom that she has, so taking care of a child can be a struggle. It is useful to remember that celebrities also deal with things like abuse, mental illness, substance use, sickness, and death. Although their wealth may provide them access to resources unavailable to most, they may still struggle in their own way. Encouraging your child to look at people who have come up with innovations and entrepreneurial ideas may be inspiring to them. It can be motivating to have big dreams, but it is also important to understand that not all realities and opportunities are granted equally. That does not mean the answer is to stop trying but to engage in the pursuit of goals with realism as well as optimism.

17. My son always wants to play video games and gets agitated if I stop him. What do I do to make this better?

Video games can stimulate the same rewards cycle response as drugs do because it activates the neural transmitter known as dopamine which is responsible for giving a pleasurable feeling.[37] [38] When you remove that pleasurable feeling associated with a drug, people can develop withdrawal symptoms that are so powerful that they are only mitigated by the next hit.[39] [40] The same phenomenon happens with video games.

I hear of children becoming physically aggressive with their caregivers when limits are attempting to be set with respect to video games. I have seen some parents just give in and allow their children to just play video games because the ensuing confrontation becomes painful and exhausting. There are resources for internet addictions and there are even burgeoning rehabilitation programs. It is also important to note that some of this can be prevented by establishing limits on video games before allowing your child access to them. Seeking outside professional help regarding this and evaluating for any underlying issue is often useful. Sometimes video games are used as escapism to avoid dealing with some other stressors. Sometimes children go through phases where are they may be immersed in video games for a while and then get tired of them. Even adults can have video game addictions which can cause stress in their interpersonal relationships, affect job functioning, and adversely affect physical health due to the sedentary nature of this activity. It is an issue that should be addressed as with any other addictive habit.

18. As a father of three girls, how do I teach them to stand up for themselves?

One way to address misogyny and patriarchy is starting at home. If you live with a female partner, do you treat her with respect and allow her to voice her opinions? A lot of men who come from patriarchal communities believe they are in fact treating the women and girls in their families well because they may be providers. Sometimes they may give respect towards the women in their family but not to their spouse. One of the first steps involves challenging your misconceptions and beliefs about gender. If you do not believe women have a place in the working world, why is that? If you believe the alternative, that they should work and contribute to providing for a household, but also should be responsible for most domestic duties, why is that? Are you at all contributing to a culture that blames women who are victims of gender discrimination or abuse?

Some of the thoughts are automatic because sociologically they have been conditioned over time. Sometimes misogyny comes in the form of getting angry when a woman challenges you in a way that might not anger you if it came from a man. In the working environment, women who ask for more are often shut down whereas the demands made by their male colleagues are honored. Look around you to see inequities around gender.

Get to know literature by women who have stood up for women's rights. Harriet Tubman is an example of a woman who risked her life to rescue so many others. If not for courageous women like her, the life of so many people would have been prematurely foreshortened. In many cultures, it is the norm for women to be oppressed, and when a man deviates from following the norm such as allowing his wife or daughter to pursue educational and professional opportunities, he is chastised and reprimanded for doing so. It then becomes easier for him to just take the path of least resistance, resulting in a cycle of oppression.

This is particularly true in environments where women are not given educational and vocational opportunities, are married off at a young age, and face gender related violence. However, the more you stand up for a woman around you, the more empowered your daughters will feel. This may mean challenging the norms of your culture, encouraging the education and professional development of your daughters, not caring what those around you will think even if they try to shame your parenting. Knowing that sometimes all it takes is one person to initiate change is a powerful reminder that doing the right thing for the future generation may benefit them immensely.

19. I am concerned about our son hanging out with a friend whose parents are millionaires. I think it will make him feel like he cannot have a better life. Should I not let him go over to their house?

Socioeconomic status can be an entity that segregates people. Social hierarchies allow for discrimination and mistreatment of those in lower socioeconomic groups in addition to racial and religious discrimination. Children should not have to be subjected to the same biases that adults may have with respect to how we view one another. Children want to play and engage in shared interests with their peers. With that said, children and adolescents do notice the differences in lifestyles and material wealth as they grow.

It can be hard for children to process why their family may not have the same things as others. Children who come from more privileged circumstances can learn to look down on children who do not come from the same privilege. I do not believe children should be segregated based on wealth. If children are lucky enough to maintain a connection, friendship and shared interests can transcend differences. You can be honest about your differences from another family, but also teach your son to be proud of his origins and feel no less than his peers. It may prove to be a valuable learning experience for both your son and his friend.

20. My 14-year-old daughter is beside herself since her boyfriend broke up with her. She cries and feels like she can never find love again. Telling her she is young and should not worry about this seems not to work. How do I help her get over this?

Young girls spend their childhood inundated with fairy tales of romantic rescues by princes on a white horse. It shapes their narrative of what expectations to have, along with what is happening in their homes. There is also an obvious underrepresentation or complete lack of representation of the LGBT and transgender communities. This may be one contributing factor as to why children who grow up in these communities feel so marginalized. It is not surprising that the damsel in distress scenario also crosses over into adulthood. I think some of this is changing with movies such as *Frozen*, which illustrates love between sisters as a type of love, although there is still a bit of a damsel in distress component in the movie as well.

There is nothing wrong with feeling that a partner can be your best friend, someone who is there for you and lifts you up. Those are all wonderful qualities to have in a partnership. However, when girls and women believe that life only really starts when they are settled with a man and children, that somehow life is not complete any other way, it impacts the ability to stay present and can impact self-esteem. There are different ways to live life and following a prescriptive pattern may just not necessarily work for everyone.

Both men and women can yearn to have support, to be taken care at times in need, and crave the companionship that can come from a stable relationship. Also, marriage is an institution seen as a commitment to possibly starting and raising a family together. When one is made to feel like a failure when they do not arrive at that destination at the right time or at all, that is a lot of people in this world being judged. Some relationships do not work out, some people are introverted and have a hard time with romantic relationships, and some do not like the idea of commitment. Part of living in a free society is that people can have their own agency, making choices about their life as they live it.

Much of our perceptions around relationships occurs by social conditioning, which starts at a young age. In the book *If Buddha Dated* by Charlotte Karl, the author describes how people often look to be taken care of in a relationship. This may be financially, emotionally, and/or physical. While a relationship should be a source of support and a platform for growth, depending on someone to be someone else's total foundation is not necessarily reasonable or even fruitful.

Interdependence should be a goal as we all need support, but neither our computer and car-driven culture of isolationistic independence or extreme codependence are necessarily the healthiest lifestyles. When a girl or woman obsesses about a man who has not called or texted her back, a therapist might gently encourage her to draw her attention back to herself and what she could do to care for herself. This is a useful thought exercise to use with your daughter when she finds herself obsessing over an ex, to encourage her to draw the attention back to herself.

She can be taught to say to herself the following: "I'm not getting what I want at this point from this person, so what can I do about it?" Sometimes, one of the hardest things to accept about rejection, as a teenager or at any age, is that people may not want anything from you. This means they may not want your friendship or a romantic relationship or anything in between. Rejection can be a painful experience.

There is an entity known as broken heart syndrome, when a part of your heart temporarily enlarges and does not pump well, while the rest of your heart functions normally or with even more forceful contractions.[41] Although usually treatable, the American Heart Association notes that broken heart syndrome can lead to severe, short-term heart muscle failure. According to social psychologist, Roy Baumeister, 98% of people have suffered from unrequited love at one time or another.[42] In a study of more than 200 incidents of unrequited love, Baumeister also found that the rejecters dealt with certain symptoms, like anxiety and guilt.[43] His study revealed that many of the pursued said things like, "I never hurt anyone before," and reported feeling bad that they had contributed to another person's pain.

Does unrequited love have an upside?[44] Lisa A. Phillips, author of *Unrequited: The Thinking Woman's Guide to Romantic Obsession*, seems to think so. "Think of all the artists, writers, and musicians who credit their achievements to a muse they couldn't win over. Van Gogh made some of his best work after Kee Vos, his beloved cousin by marriage, broke his heart. Dante fell in love with Beatrice when he was eight, and as an adult immortalized his devotion to her in La Vita Nuova and The Divine Comedy. In the wake of romantic rejection, legendary dancer Isadora Duncan had a crucial epiphany about her approach to movement. As she wrote in her autobiography, she directed her emotions 'toward my art, which gave me the joys which love withheld.' In our own time, Smith, Adele, and Taylor Swift are giving voice to unrequited love in their music."

Phillips goes on to say that, "Creative inspiration isn't the only positive outcome of romantic rejection. More than a third of the 260 women I surveyed for my book reported that the experience 'changed my life for the better.' Some credited their unrequited feelings with pushing them to leave fizzling marriages, begin their lives anew in another state, come out or learn a new language. Because desire, as one Jungian analyst recently described it to me, gives us a sense of possibility, it may help us see what's missing in our lives."

Love can be one of the greatest sources of mental energy. Neuroscience research has shown there is an actual neurochemical response that is otherwise known as the falling in love phenomenon. Dopamine is released and provides a "high," mimicking the response that is experienced with drugs.[45] This feeling is so addictive and feels vital to being. Other chemicals involved include serotonin, which elevates mood, oxytocin, which promotes bonding, and endorphins, which are responsible for pleasure sensations.[46]

Unfortunately, this neurochemical reaction also results in people going against their better judgment. An otherwise law-abiding citizen can end up with someone with a criminal record. This is exaggerated in adolescents who go through a certain developmental stage of neurodevelopment. During this time, they are more likely to take risks and be more impulsive. They are less likely to utilize sound judgment and employ problem-solving skills.[47] [48] This is also a period of experimentation. These neurochemical reactions have played an evolutionary role in propagating species. They are part of the instinctual drive in the animal kingdom, which results in mating behavior necessary for procreation. This reaction eventually decreases over a period of 18 to 24 months.[49][50] This is possibly why it takes so long for a person to get over someone. Understanding the neurochemical reaction can put things in perspective and help to evaluate rationally if this is a person who is genuinely good for you. The benefit of the reaction is that it can foster good relationship bonding and serve as a warm reminder of attachment during rough times. This can help a couple work through differences and keep a family together with the focus on healthy dynamics. As a result, the effects can be positive.

The downside of this very same neurochemical reaction is that in can result in one choosing to stay in a bad relationship where there is mistreatment and holding on too long to something deleterious. Love can cause feelings of euphoria or result in following the feeling into potentially unhealthy situations. Perhaps we can use this knowledge to make better choices and teach our children to also do so. We can keep in mind that although "falling in love" is powerful, we should also notice character strengths, such as emotional generosity and kindness. Physical attraction is one type of attraction, but other ones can be equally rewarding, such as shared goals and values. Many of us are fortunate to have choices in this area, but much of the world does not have the freedom of choice, particularly in oppressive communities.

The adage of using both your head and your heart can mean more than a cliché in this realm. I think this situation can be used as an opportunity to help your daughter understand her feelings and why she is struggling to move on. If she learns how to view her emotions more objectively, it may help her make better romantic decisions in the future and to know what qualities to look for in a partner. Adolescents and young adults are not given guidelines or taught how to handle romantic rejection in school. Romantic attraction and connection are part of development, and it would be helpful if we paid attention to how to help people navigate confusing feelings.

21. I worry that my 13-year-old daughter is growing up taking things for granted living a more privileged life than I had. How do I teach her humility?

My father used to talk to me a lot when I was younger about not having too much attachment to material things, stating that an enlightened mind is a much more desirable asset. There are some elements of lifestyle choices children pick up from the families they grow up in. If you can take nice trips and ride in nicer vehicles than you did in your childhood but want to teach your children similar simplistic values, think about how you can do that realistically.

When I was a teenager, my family took a trip to India and my parents made us take crowded public buses everywhere instead of cars or even autos which offered a little more privacy. The goal was to teach us what it would be like if were to live with more simplistic means. Unfortunately, after a bad incident right at the beginning of the trip where a man groped me on the bus, the whole appreciation of what my parents were getting at became lost to me.

I simply just longed to get back to the comforts of my U.S. lifestyle, with air conditioning and modern bathrooms. I do not fault my parents for wanting me to incorporate a more simplistic life, however. You can moderate how much expendable cash you allow your daughter to have and encourage her to volunteer with those less fortunate. Doing that can offer her some perspective. Reading books and watching documentaries to teach her about how others are faring in less fortunate and often perilous circumstances can also offer perspective.

22. My boyfriend yells at me constantly in front of my teenage son. What will this do to him? How do I deal with this?

Watching this can create stress and anxiety in your son. It can cause him to be distracted from schoolwork, cause feelings of restlessness, irritability, other symptoms of depression. Also, he can feel helpless in terms of being able to protect you. You may suffer the consequences of being verbally abused as well, some of the same symptoms, as well as a decrease in self-esteem, lack of control, stress, depression, and anxiety.[51] It can also be hard to leave these situations, but they can be psychologically and medically jeopardous to you and your son. Getting outside help can help you empower yourself to gain the strength to deal with this. If you want to stay with your boyfriend, couples therapy is recommended to work out this dynamic. If he is not willing and is not interested in change, it is probably best to leave such a relationship. Some women stay in a relationship for financial reasons, etc., so figuring out ways to empower yourself can help you make a good decision.

23. My child is smart, but his grades do not reflect that. He is failing two classes and does not seem to care, so how do I make him care? After all, his whole future is at stake!

This is a question I get a lot from parents. They feel frustrated that they cannot make their child pay attention and care about their academic performances. Sometimes, children feel rebellious. A little bit of this is to be expected, as years of schooling can be tedious and mundane, causing frustration on the part of the child. When a child is struggling academically, they can become demoralized and lose confidence in their ability. Tutoring can help a child and working together with the school on evaluation for any learning-related issues can be helpful.

In the U.S., an evaluation for an individualized education plan can be requested to allow for accommodations in the classroom. Sometimes lack of motivation can be related to an underlying issue such as depression, anxiety, reaction to stress at home. Excessive pressure can result in stress and affect motivation. Chastising the child or humiliating them is not a good approach to dealing with this situation. Instead, taking an approach of inquiry may be more productive. Perhaps your child does not have a good connection with a particular teacher, or the teaching style is not one that resonates with your child. Some children have Attention Deficit Hyperactivity Disorder, which can affect focus and attention. These are things that should be evaluated for if they are a concern by a trained mental health specialist.

Substance use is also something that can affect school performance and parents may be unaware that this going on. Inhalant use can develop into an addiction and easy to access in canisters of items like whipping cream. There can be any number of reasons that a child has difficulty with school. Sometimes children become bored and uninterested, some feel burned out with the repetitive nature of studying and exams. The amount of external pressure to succeed may need to be mitigated to foster providing encouragement, rather than having a counterproductive effect with excessive pressure.

24. My 14-year-old son gets extremely angry when he is confronted about anything. He leaves the house without permission, and I worry that he is possibly using substances to deal with his emotions. How do I help him with his anger?

Anger can be result of stress, trauma, or a combination of genetic and environmental influences. Since teenagers become their own autonomous individuals that are growing, it is during this time where many parents feel they are unable to influence the child's behavior or have a sense of control over some of their child's judgment. Sometimes children express anger when they are feeling depressed or irritated and it can be a sign of an underlying mental illness. Substance use can cause erratic mood changes and explosive behavior. Teenagers can become agitated when they are withdrawing from substances and apparently not realize that this is happening. Sometimes a young person may use substances to self-medicate intense emotions that are overwhelming to deal with. Finding out whether there are stressors that you do not know about can clarify the origins your teens emotional responses. They should have someone they can talk to like a therapist who can help them navigate these emotions and find better ways of coping. External limit setting such as limiting available funds and appropriate supervision may help mitigate risk of substance use.

However, sometimes more intensive interventions are required if the teen becomes a danger to him or herself or to others in the home. When explosive behavior cannot be controlled, evaluation by emergency mental health professionals who respond to crisis situations maybe warranted. Sometimes entities like law enforcement may need to be called to prevent further harm, but ideally a mental health professional trained in crisis care should also be involved. Of course, the availability of such personnel varies all over the world and sometimes is completely nonexistent. A parent should not feel disempowered by a teenager who exhibits this kind of behavior. If it is ongoing behavior, inpatient treatment or an alternative placement may have to be considered as an option. There are residential treatment facilities that can be an option for teenagers with ongoing aggression. This also depends on geographical availability, insurance coverage, and other compounding factors such as quality of care.

Sometimes medication can help with explosive behavior even if it is considered a shorter short-term option. If substance abuse is part of the picture than treatment for that is needed. I have had patients who come from different cultural backgrounds and are reacting to oppression by exhibiting anger and explosiveness. For example, teenage girls who are worried that their parents are going to marry them at a young age to a stranger without their consent can react in such a fashion to rebel. This is completely understandable as well as a healthy response, and the focus should instead be on how to address the well-being of the young girl and stand up against potentially harmful cultural practices. Physical discipline may only increase aggressive behaviors in young people so that is not advised unless if it is solely in self-defense where restraint or techniques may be needed to avoid danger to others.

25. My husband is leaving me for another woman. What will this teach my daughters?

One of the things we begin to understand as we mature is that some things in life are not under our control. Whether it is a job layoff from a company that is downsizing, a romantic rejection, or unexpected illness, these things can be a source of grief. When you are dealing with a crumbling marriage whether it is from adultery or other issues, you often go through a process of grief. Occasionally, some people feel relieved at the end of a marriage, but there is usually quite a bit of pain involved during the process. What makes it harder is considering the ramifications for your children.

The concept of parents separating can be stressful for children and teens. A therapist of any kind will tell you that one of the worst things you can do is disparage the other parent in front of your child. This is because the child's identity comes from both parents, and it can affect his or her self-esteem. If a child observes unpleasant interactions, a better way of talking about it might be something like this: "I am sorry you saw your parents arguing. We should not have done that in front of you. We try not to but sometimes we mess up."

Children and teenagers can be way more perceptive than we give them credit for. You would be surprised at how much children know and what they disclose to me about their parents' marriages. They often know details of infidelity, hurtful names either parent calls the other, and the specifics of what their parents argue about. Concerning adultery or any type of betrayal, a child may feel inclined to be protective of the parent who feels they were wronged. Often, a child is encouraged to pick a side and or acts out with the other parent as a show of solidarity with one parent. A child may also feel guilty for secretly being relieved and happy for the parent who moved on with someone else. This may be because it was difficult to be around people who did not get along with each other, or they feel closer and more bonded with the unfaithful parent.

Another question I often get asked about is what this does to a child's ability to trust adults in the future, the effect on their own beliefs regarding commitment, and their ability to cope. It is loaded, no matter how you slice it. The answer is complicated, affected by a child's natural resilience, changes in the environment, the child's temperament, and psychological makeup, as well as genetics. Research shows us it is not the conflict itself but how the conflict is dealt with that predicts future outcomes.[52]

Children who experienced acrimonious parental relationships can have difficulty in trusting adult relationships. They may reenact some of the trauma they experienced, such as choosing someone to get involved with who ends up being unfaithful and causes pain. This is not something they may consciously know and certainly, it is not helpful to blame them, but sometimes we are drawn to what is familiar. However, many children grow up to have healthy relationships and cope quite well.

It is important to understand your daughter's developmental stage. A child is not a friend with who you can discuss in detail all your anger and hurt about your spouse. It is not helpful for your child to hear you blame your spouse for ruining your life. It is not helpful for your child to hear you plot revenge. "Hell hath no fury like a woman scorned," William Congreve said in *The Morning Bride*. You can feel it, but you must understand that certain conversations are not appropriate to have with children. They should be reserved for adults or therapists. If a child finds out about adultery, which may be inevitable and hard to conceal, especially if the other parent brings their new partner into the child's life, it is important that the child feels they can talk about it and express themselves.

You do not want to raise your daughter to think that you are a victim and that all men are bad and cannot be trusted. It is important to role model emotional self-reliance and healthy coping skills. It may be impossible to completely conceal your grief, but reassurance helps.

"Mommy is going through a bit of a rough time right now because of the problems I had with your dad. I am sorry if you see me cry sometimes or seem sad. I want you to know that it will get better and that I am working on dealing with it while being a good mom for you."

If a child sees their parents gracefully handle adversity, it will probably help them navigate rough times. I have seen young girls come into my office repeating some of the sentiments of their scorned mothers, such as that they do not believe you can trust a man, that they do not believe in marriage or commitment, and that they should just focus on other things. This is also true if the tables are turned, and the father is the one being scorned. I have seen boys who see their mother being disrespected and are taught it is okay to do that.

You do not want to paint a dark and gloomy picture of the future for your children. You want to help them think positively and to learn to be discerning but also to trust certain people. Sometimes, even when there is adultery, couples have restored their relationship, often with the help of counseling. This is a personal decision only you can make, sometimes with the help of a therapist. Unfortunately, when parents do reconcile, the parent who feels victimized can bring it up repeatedly in front of the children which does not benefit the children. In that case, you can end up re-exposing your kids to your pain.

If reconciliation is in the works, establish ground rules with your partner about letting the past go, especially in front of your children. Your children are individuals, you foray your process of healing and need to be mindful not to project your emotional issues and difficulties onto them. This can be a tall order as the grieving process is not always easy to do in private, and children pick up on their parents' stress. Just acknowledging to yourself that you are going through a hard time, showing yourself self-compassion, can be the first step in showing compassion for your children's journey.

······●●●●●●●●●······

PART FOUR

LATE ADOLESCENCE AND YOUNG ADULTS

15 TO 21 YEARS

1. My daughter wants to take a gap year after graduating high school this year. I think this will cause her to lose focus, so how do I approach this?

Many high school students consider the idea of taking a gap year. This varies across cultures. For example, it is typical for many students in Australia and New Zealand to take a year after finishing high school to travel the world before beginning university studies. It is also glaringly obvious that a gap year is not affordable to many minority kids in urban communities. High school is the time to have frank discussions with teenagers about finances and how higher education can be funded. Be transparent about any limitations without making your kids worry about how much you can or cannot contribute.

Some parents struggle with health issues or a lack of opportunity to earn the income necessary to help their children with their education. Some teenagers must contribute to caretaking aging grandparents or other family members, and that role can last well into adulthood. Life circumstances make a big impact on education-related decisions. Many teenagers in urban and rural communities feel that they must begin working as soon as they finish school or even before so they can contribute to family finances. This is vastly different from students in more affluent suburban communities who come from families with more available resources.

Even with resource limitations, you can help your children find ways to actualize academic dreams. There are different ways of looking at a gap year. It can be a meaningful time in life. There are numerous humanitarian and wildlife organizations that offer volunteer opportunities worldwide, some with accommodations and stipends for basic expenses. Some people join the Peace Corps. A gap year can allow a teenager to broaden their perspectives in different parts of the world as they enter adulthood.

It also does not have to involve traveling, especially at this time during a pandemic, and traveling is broadly cautioned against. There are many opportunities in the U.S., which include paid employment or volunteer work. It can be a time to pursue mindfulness activities, too, such as meditation and yoga. These can be profoundly moving experiences that are centering and rejuvenating. A gap year may also address the issue of a student entering college "crispy," which essentially means a teenager who feels burned out from being overwhelmed with the workload and activities of primary school education before he or she even enters college.

Is it also possible that your child stays home for a year without much productivity? Will idle time affect motivation? Could the free time expose them to drugs and alcohol to deal with boredom? Is it possible that they lose their interest in higher education? Yes, these things are possibilities that do warrant consideration. The other possibility is that many people use the time in a way they end up being challenged and learn valuable lessons while expending their energy in different ways. These are useful discussions to have with your daughter.

Is it possible that a college may have been easier to get into without taking a gap year? That varies according to the university and field of study. Sometimes, adding new experiences to a resume can helps an application. A gap year can also happen anytime. It can be useful to find out what your daughter might want to do later as well. For example, living in another country and picking up another language can be useful for future job prospects. My time in India was valuable in helping me understand people with different backgrounds. Young people should be able to know that there is life beyond their neighborhood.

Being on in certain academic tracks that involve intensive training later may not allow the opportunity to break away for a year and come back to it. The same applies to adults in various careers. Many parents do not feel like they can take a gap year abroad while raising a child and many do not feel they can take time off from their jobs, as they must financially support their families. It may help to facilitate an exercise where your daughter writes down a plan for how she would hypothetically divide her time and what she would do. Be clear about how much you will be involved, whether it is financially feasible, etc. As adults, most of us often dream about what we would do if we had a year off to do anything we wanted. Some of us would write a book or two. Hearing about your daughter's experiences of discovery as she grows can be heartwarming and allow you to reflect on pursuing some of your own passions.

2. Our 16-year-old son was attacked on his way home from school. We reported this to the police but now he is afraid to go outside or even go to class. How do we help them feel safe?

This is something a lot of parents worry about when they allow their children some independence, will it put them in danger? Walking to and from school is an experience that children should be able to do safely but unfortunately in many parts of the world, going to school is fraught with dangers. It is not uncommon after such an event for a child to be scared and anxious, even if the perpetrators were apprehended. If there are ongoing reports of violence in the area, that can limit your teen's ability to feel a sense of control over his safety, not to mention also cause worrying as a parent. He may benefit from having someone accompany him on his commute and therapy to help deal with his anxiety.

Anxiety happens when our bodies sense danger, which can be protective. However, when it escalates, it can affect functioning. People who have experienced trauma may develop symptoms of acute stress disorder or posttraumatic stress disorder. This includes experiencing flashbacks, nightmares, hyper vigilance, irritability, and worrying about bad things happening or a foreshortened future. Sometimes symptoms can be severe, interrupting sleep, and they can wax and wane for many years. For some people, medication can help manage some of the symptoms. Exposure therapy which is involves revisiting the area where the trauma happened can take place gradually with the help of an experienced therapist. If it is an area with ongoing violence, that may not be possible.

Some communities have neighborhood watchdog patrols where security is monitored by designated people who drive around. However, in the U.S., this has also resulted in racial profiling, death of African Americans after being wrongfully targeted, so this is a complicated issue needing the eradication of explicit and implicit biases. Discussing with the school staff ways to keep the students safe and whether there is a counselor available who can check in on your son can also help to manage his anxiety.

3. My spouse has repeatedly put me down in front of our children. I want to snap back at her but do not want to upset the kids, so I do not say anything. How do I teach her that it is important to treat me with respect for so many reasons, including role modeling for our children even as they are now older?

Demeaning the other parent in front of children is not only hurtful, it also does not model healthy behaviors in front of children. Remarks that are cutting and bring another person down such occur in the form of criticism and sarcasm. That is kind of language can be very damaging to a relationship because overtime the roads it erodes on a person's self-esteem, disempowering them. It also does not feel good to be put down in front of your children and can teach your children not to treat you with respect. One way to address this behavior is by having a conversation with her away from the children, explaining to her what you notice is happening, and how it makes you feel.

Sometimes a spouse is not aware of what they are doing and the ramifications it has on children. You can ask her to be mindful of this language. Engage in couples therapy if needed to work things out. If the behavior does not change, this may be damaging to your marriage and your children. Some of the comments your partner may have felt it was made in jest. For example, when stereotypical gender roles are not filled such as when the man is not handy around the house with fixing things or happens to become fearful when he sees a spider. Your partner may feel that they were just making a joke because they found it amusing. When it begins to feel demeaning or humiliating, that could mean it something more pervasive. This can be tricky because different people can be sensitive to different things, laughing at one joke but feeling hurt by another. It is important that there is healthy communication about these things.

A partner repeatedly telling you that you are not a man because you do not make enough money to buy nice things, or that you are not manly in other ways to humiliate you is not healthy. This kind of behavior can be insidious over time and cause a rift that is irreparable. This is worth trying to address this early on. Sometimes change is possible when a certain degree of emotional intelligence and maturity exists, and sometimes it is not. A man who takes pride in being a househusband, participating in child-rearing, doing domestic duties if he is not the breadwinner in the family, should not have to feel emasculated if it is a partnership that works for both of you. If you can flourish in certain ways like with professional ambition (if that is important to you) by having a supportive partner who manages other responsibilities, that can be fulfilling. Often one partner can resent the other partner when they are not contributing equally to the relationship, and this can accumulate resentment and anger. Learning to communicate and work together can build closeness as well mutual support.

4. When my 15-year-old daughter casually brought up a question about birth control with me I was shocked and concerned. I do not want her to be sexually active, so how do I stop her from doing this?

It is a good thing for teenagers to know about birth control and means of protecting themselves. One of the ways you can protect your daughter with respect to sexual activity is by having an open conversation about this without shaming. Speaking of sex as sinful or other negative ways can also affect future perceptions around normal human intimacy so it is useful to understand that. Explaining to her the risks such as sexually transmitted diseases, unwanted pregnancies, and not having the emotional bandwidth yet to deal with complicated feelings that arise from sexual activity at a young age can be useful conversations to have.

It is important to talk to her about how she and her body should be treated with respect. Exposure to drugs, alcohol, and sex can happen when young people are not appropriately supervised, and even in the most sheltered families where there is lots of supervision. Some clever teenagers sneak out at night without their parents knowing. If you do not know where your child is or what they are engaged in, they are left to navigate potentially risky behavior and can be vulnerable to predators. Different sets of parents and cultures have different belief systems about how sheltered life they want their teenagers to live until they become adults. In many cultures that are oppressive to women, that even continues throughout adulthood.

You may not be able to control the entirety of your teenage daughter's behaviors, but you can make sure she has the information to make sound judgments about sexual activity. If she decides to engage in it, she at least has information about how to keep herself safe. The human papillomavirus (HPV) vaccine is recommended to help prevent future infections in young people that can lead to other complications like cervical cancer.[1]

If you do not feel comfortable, make sure your child can talk to a doctor or another authority who can provide her with information about safe sexual activity. Young people need to know this information before they engage in sexual activity. It does not mean that just because they have the information, they are going to begin to be reckless. Discussing the benefits of abstinence at a young age can help your daughter become aware of the choices she has concerning protecting her body and warding off unwanted consequences. Hormonal changes bring about different feelings in the body and it can be confusing to know how to respond as a young person.

I do meet teenagers who want to have a child for different reasons, whether it is to escape a home they are unhappy in by creating another family, having an ailing parent, and wanting to bring them joy, or a simply a matter of thinking it would be a nice experience to have a baby. This is usually an ill-informed decision that is not made with understanding all the future ramifications of an early pregnancy, but it happens. In some communities it is even encouraged. You want to give your teens knowledge and improve their understanding of the possibilities of different choices. Knowing the potential benefits of waiting can help them choose wisely.

5. We have three kids at home, ages 15, 17, and 19. My husband does not believe we need to eat together as a family at dinner time. He will take his plate into the living room and watch TV. I feel this is a loss of valuable bonding time with our kids. How do I change this?

A lot of parents are not aware of how valuable bonding time can be lost during the sharing of more routine aspects of life. With the advent of technological devices, it is not uncommon for the whole family to be distracted and not engage socially. Alternatively, your husband may believe that time is also valuable "me time" where he gets to decompress and relax. Parents can disagree on how time with family should be spent and what moments should be capitalized on.

Many people grow up having fond memories of eating meals with family and having it a time where they can talk about one another's day. He may agree with you on this or may feel he spends enough time with the family during other moments. If he continues to refuse, consider whether he finds time to connect with the family at other times. If so, then maybe that is a perspective worth noting. Many couples also do not agree on the amount or what is quality time with their children.

When it comes to raising children, one of the challenges many couples face is agreeing on certain values. Parents can argue about what snacks they should feed their children if they feel hungry or how much screen time should be permissible. In this case, you see dinnertime as a valuable resource that can be utilized to promote family bonding and closeness. Either your husband does not believe the same thing, or he does not prioritize it the way you do. He also may simply not think of it as a missed opportunity.

One way of addressing this is to first have a discussion with him when you are both relaxed and away from the children. The first step would be having a talk with him explaining that you feel that mealtime would be a valuable time for bonding with family as it is a natural break in the day. You can explain your feelings about this and why you think it is important for your family to spend time this way. He may respond that he feels he spends plenty of time with the family and this is a time to decompress after a long day. We need to recognize something as a problem before we can ever change it. Perhaps you both can agree on your husband joining some of the family dinners where he is fully present. Afterwards you can check in with him on what that is like for him.

Habits are often hard to break, and they often take a long time to change. A person also needs to feel an internal motivation to want to change, seeing the value in making change happen. If he is not bothered by it, it can take time for a person to realize how they are impacting others and whether that warrants a need for change. The goal to work towards would be that you come to a mutual agreement on what is acceptable.

Getting someone to do something simply because you want them, is not the most effective strategy. Marshall Rosenberg, in his book *Nonviolent Communication* (A Language of Life), encourages a collaborative process of communication where you connect with the other person in an empathic way that leads to sharing of thoughts and ideas but understanding that the other person has their freedom of choices.

If it turns out that your husband does not want to change or see the value of change, then you may have to make peace with it. Maybe you can agree on other activities he would prefer to share with the family. Perhaps he can be the one who reads to your children or bonds with your children in other ways, taking them on picnics or other outings. This may not feel the same as a shared family dinner, but it may result in a situation you are both satisfied with if you have been trying to force family mealtime when one person is not participating.

You can also want to enjoy time with your children, even if done independently from your husband. Perhaps he joins the family for a walk after dinner. I once read a story about a family who takes after-dinner walks every day. Even after the children became adults, whenever they would visit home, the family continued their evening strolls. The whole family cherished those moments. It might be useful to focus your attention on things that your husband does do for the children, to help keep some perspective.

Maybe he is supportive of your children's dreams and drives them around to sports practices and recitals. Maybe he is gentle in his approach and has a lot of patience. He may be hard worker and a provider so to him, he may feel that this is how he shows his love. I understand that you do not want him to miss out on special moments and opportunities for bonding since children grow up so quickly. You can gently help him come to that realization by communication and encouragement. Otherwise, you may want to focus on what is working and treasure it.

6. How do I stop my 15-year-old son from texting and driving? I am terrified he will be distracted one day on the road from looking at his phone and get into an accident.

Cell phones unfortunately are the cause of many accidents because they are distracting. They can cause drivers to not focus on the road and it can decrease reaction time if they are distracted.[2] One way to deal with this is to set up notifications on the cell phone where a "do not disturb message" pops up in response to messages when you are driving, or your son is driving. That prevents the phone from stimulating him to look at it when he receives a text message.

However, a notification message to others may still not stop him from looking at the phone. It is important to discuss safety concerns such as cell phone distraction with your son to prevent future accidents. You can have him watch public service announcements about texting and driving and find out about informational campaigns focused on educating teenagers about this. Helping you develop good habits to keep him safe on the road may minimize the risk of accidents.

Some cars come with automatic safety brakes and alerts that may help with driving safety. Using a device that holds the cell phone when your son needs to glance at it for GPS directions can prevent the distraction of him looking downwards. Public service announcements can be powerful tools to help young people understand the dangers. It can be powerful to hear from parents who lost a child from a texting related accident involving a cell phone. Some grieving parents speak to young people either in person or through virtual platforms to help prevent other parents from experiencing the same type of pain. There are educational resources available to teach teens about safety while driving worth looking into. It is not only young people who get distracted, adults get distracted by cell phones when they are driving. Therefore, it may be prudent for adults to review some of this information as well.

7. My 16-year-old daughter wants to be addressed as "they." I am having a rough time with doing this as I think she is a girl. How do I deal with this?

If you are having a tough time with this, imagine that it is probably more difficult for your daughter to share this with you. Gender dysphoria is when a young person is uncomfortable with their biological sex, causing uncomfortable feelings of sadness and despair. Having the experience of feeling like a boy in girl's body can be very painful emotionally and even result in depression and suicidal thoughts.[3] It is understandable to have concerns if your child identifies as another gender. Transgender individuals are discriminated against worldwide and many of them have been killed in hate crimes. Finding communities where they fit in or feel accepted can be a big challenge. They also deal with being shunned by others.

The US government under the order of the Trump administration tried to ban transgender individuals from military services, which would also be denying them benefits and pensions. This represents a form of discrimination along with other measures such as eliminating them from census data is like the dangers of racism or religious bigotry. It would be a good idea for your child to see a therapist who understands what your child is experiencing and can help you accept and support this journey.

Chastising or humiliating your child, refusing to use the pronoun of choice, or altogether disowning your child can be devastating for a young person. Remember this is not simply a matter of choosing a certain lifestyle, it is more complicated. You can create a nurturing and supportive environment that helps your child thrive. It may not look the way you anticipated but the bond of love between you and your child can continue to grow despite that. It may expand your compassion and ability to accept others as well. Do not run away from your child's emotional process because your child needs you now more than ever.

It is natural to worry about how your child will be treated others, but also do not let your concern over other's opinions cloud what may be in the best interest of your child's health. Your child's health and happiness are more important than the gossiping, judgmental people that try to cultivate a toxic environment of shame. Focus on what is important. It does not mean your child cannot achieve dreams or find a place in this world that feels like home. As a parent, you are responsible for sensible guidance with the knowledge that your child will have their own free will as an adult(hopefully).

People can have questions about their gender association and sexuality at different times in life. Sometimes it is transitory, sometimes there is a strong urge to want to change gender and even undertake sexual gender reassignment surgery. Some parents ask themselves if they did something wrong or is this a result of some type of trauma their child experienced when they were young. It may very well be neither of those things, your child may just identify more with a specific pronoun and may have questions about their gender. Children navigate their own experience in this world, and they need you to support their emotional journey even if there are parts of the journey that troubles you.

8. I found pornography on my son's laptop; I am terrified he is heading in a bad direction. What can I do? I do not want to embarrass him to the extent that he will not talk to me about things.

It is normal for your son to have a curiosity about sex and sexual activity. In the past, teenage boys would find depictions of sexual activity in magazines as film depictions would often be restricted but overtime the access to pornography through digital devices has increased. You do not want to embarrass or shame him for this, but you do want to set limits on this type of behavior because it can have some ramifications. Depending on the amount and frequency of pornographic consumption, it can set up unrealistic expectations of what sex should be like, and it can show examples of mistreatment. It can also become addictive because it can stimulate the reward center of the brain.[4]

You can set up parenting controls on digital devices that your son uses and talk to him openly about the ramifications without making him feel humiliated. You can set limits, and let it be known that you do not want him taking in this content because you are concerned about how it can affect him. Younger children should not be exposed to adult themes as they may not be able to process it, can interpret it as something violent, and it may lead to precious sexual activity in the future. You also do not want your son to develop a demeaning attitude about women by repeatedly watching this content. Therefore, it is entirely appropriate to set limits and try to redirect his attention. You may not be able to control every type of stimulation he receives from outside sources, but you can help promote the concept of a healthy curiosity around sexual fantasy. There are sex education experts that speak in schools to students about this and answer questions in a safe space.

9. My 17-year-old daughter washes her hands about 50 times a day. How do I stop her from doing this so much? Why does she do this?

Obsessive-compulsive disorder (OCD) is a type of anxiety disorder where there are obsessions about various topics like germs. The obsessions cause one to engage in compulsive behavior. For example, the fear of germs or the fear of getting sick may be causing your daughter to wash her hands so many times. With the COVID-19 pandemic, symptoms of OCD can be exacerbated in individuals who suffer from them, and there are some symptoms that can also develop in people who do not have a history of an anxiety disorder or OCD.[5] Hand washing is a public health measure that has been encouraged to limit the spread of COVID-19, and this can be triggering to those suffering from OCD.

A skilled therapist can help guide your daughter in dealing with this. Cognitive-behavioral therapy can help reframe obsessive thoughts and limit compulsive behavior.[6] Part of cognitive therapy can involve exposure therapy which can help to alleviate obsessive-compulsive symptoms.[7] Many people can learn to manage their symptoms in a way that does not affect their daily functioning too much. For many high-performing people, their OCD becomes functional in a way at their jobs because their attention to detail is beneficial. However, it can prevent experiencing joy when the focus is on perfection and cause irritability, dissatisfaction, self-blame. When it becomes paralyzing or impacts functioning, whether it is academic, professional, or interpersonal relationships, then it is a good idea to seek treatment. Sometimes OCD is problematic enough and does not respond to therapy without some medication management. That is something to be discussed with a doctor who is comfortable treating OCD.

10. My 18-year-old daughter just told me she is pregnant and is planning to move in with her boyfriend who is 19. She wants to keep the pregnancy. I am angry and devastated because this shatters the dreams, I had for her. What do I do now?

It is natural for parents to have hopes and dreams for their children, along with a desire to protect them from whimsical decisions that can affect their life in a negative way. In this case, you do have legitimate reason for concern. Pregnancies can make people feel incredibly joyful, or shocked, and devastated, depending on the culture, ages of the prospective mother and father, timing, and other factors. In some cultures, early pregnancy is welcome. In some situations, there is a built-in acceptance that the father may or may not be part of the child's life, and that he may or may not commit to the mother.

Research shows that when prospective parents are further along in their education, such as having a college degree had less stress, and were less anxious about parenting.[8] Women with less education were also found to experience more stress while parenting.[9] As a parent of a pregnant young adult barely out of her teenage years, you may experience a lot of concerns. You may think that your daughter and her boyfriend are too young, and not ready for this kind of responsibility. You also probably understand that there may be a lack of emotional maturity. If the parents' relationship is not healthy or there is mistreatment, it is possible that the child may suffer some trauma. You may also have an opinion about the readiness of the father. These concerns are all valid and it is understandable why you feel disappointed and deeply worried.

One thing that is hard to accept is that you may not be able to control the choices your daughter makes. You may simultaneously want to rescue her, but also think that you do not want to take on additional parenting simply because you do not believe your daughter and boyfriend will be responsible parents. You might just want to be a grandparent who enjoys your time with a grandchild instead of having to take an active, essential role in raising your grandchild.

Some parents in your situation may feel the urge to disown their child for becoming pregnant so young, and they may also have mixed feelings about also wanting to embrace the joy that comes with having a grandchild. Eventually, some forgiveness is required for all parties. You may need to forgive your daughter for jumping into this role before you thought she was ready. You may need to forgive yourself for feeling that you were not able to prevent it.

If your daughter decides to carry on with her pregnancy, it is useful to start imagining what possibilities and resources may exist to support her. For a lot of people who have children young, they may be able to return to pursuing their educational goals later. I have friends who have earned graduate degrees while raising children. They may have to work hard while trying to juggle childcare, which can be challenging, but these are personal choices to make.

Sometimes, people wait until their children are older and more independent before focusing on some academic or professional goals, instead choosing a vocation to meet financial needs for the time being. For many young parents, financial stability can be hard to come by, so they do not ever feel that pursuing higher educational goals can be a possibility. Other parents may have underlying challenges like a learning disability which caused them to lose confidence in their abilities and may have even motivated them to find fulfillment by becoming a parent.

I have seen that for some young women who become pregnant, having a child gives them a new sense of purpose in their life which can be grounding. For some, it motivated them to give up an unhealthy partying lifestyle, reckless behavior, and to live with more intention. This is by no means an endorsement for early pregnancy. There are clear benefits to waiting a while, but we must recognize that you do not have to look at it as the end of your daughter's potential in life.

Many successful leaders, politicians, professors, and doctors are women who had children at a young age and then navigated their professional aspirations over time. Support groups and nonprofit organizations can help you and your daughter through this experience if there are available services for young mothers. She may qualify for certain resources that will help her get quality healthcare, including mental health care. This can help new parents create a safe, loving, and nurturing environment for their children. It may not be the exact vision you imagined for her, but she may end up crafting a life that works for her family.

11. I am worried about my teenage son's friends because they do not seem like good company. What do I do about this?

It is useful to understand why you think this. Do you know if they are using substances or involved in illegal activity such as stealing or other behaviors? Do you have any preconceived notions about people of different backgrounds or socioeconomic statuses that are influencing your opinion? On the same note, do you assume that people coming from the same backgrounds are necessarily good influences?

Sometimes your intuition is correct in that there can be harmful influences that direct a child into unhealthy behaviors. If they are surrounded by company that engages in skipping school and failing classes by not exhibiting any academic effort, that may not be a good influence for your child. If his friends use substances, there may be a lot of peer pressure for him to do the same. Sometimes when teenagers feel emotional pain, they connect with other teenagers who are also experiencing pain and react to it in maladaptive ways.

For example, a teenager who deals with depression may feel comfortable sharing their emotions with someone else who deals with depression. You may feel like this is harmful because it does not challenge them to harness another perspective to lift your child out of depression. There can also be a codependency that develops in the relationship that may not be healthy for either teenager. This can also happen in adult relationships.

However, some of the friends that you do not approve of may be solid support systems for your child and may be the ones that show up when your child needs a good friend. Sometimes when you pressure your child to be friends with those who you think are good examples, that does not mean that the relationship becomes automatically a healthy one. Even though you feel that the child who is succeeding is a better influence, those children can also be bullies and unhealthy influences in certain ways. Sometimes high functioning children can be involved with substance use and other behaviors that adults are not aware of.

You can talk to your son about your concerns about some of his friends and why feel that. You do have the right and responsibility to provide appropriate supervision, which can minimize the prospect that he is influenced in a negative way. Getting your son involved in sports or other pro-social activities can keep him engaged with people who may be healthier influences. You do not want to compare your son to others and say to him "why can't you be more like this person." It is reasonable to highlight good qualities such as empathy, politeness, a strong work ethic when you see it in others, but you should also acknowledge your son's good qualities. Coming home to a nurturing environment where his parents are understanding and supportive will help your son build a foundation where he can choose wisely when it comes to friendships.

12. We went as a family to a New Year's party where parents were giving their children sips of alcohol. I do not believe there is any need to introduce kids to this and do not understand the argument that it quells their curiosity. Should I skip these parties from now on?

In general, alcohol use in children can affect the developing brain.[10] [11] However, many parents feel giving their child a few sips here and there is not harmful and satisfies their curiosity about alcohol. You do not have to have the same beliefs as other parents, and you can have a different view as my parents did. My parents did not allow any alcohol exposure and I did not have my first sip until after my 21st birthday when it was legal to do so. Fortunately for me, I have never loved the taste of alcohol, so I do not crave it in the way others do and never developed a desire to drink frequently or heavily.

You can give your child some sparkling water or cider instead of alcohol saying that you do not want your child to drink it. You can stand by your decision and explain that you have different views about this than some of other parents, and that is okay. If it does make you consistently uncomfortable you could skip the parties in the future. These are value systems that people have different opinions about. In certain religions like Judaism, alcohol is given to young people as part of a religious ritual. In other religions such as Islam, alcohol is forbidden so there is not even a question of exposure at a young age if the family follows their faith. In Hinduism, devotees are encouraged not to engage in behaviors that are harmful to themselves or others and alcohol does not have a religious significance.

Some parents think that allowing their teenagers to drink at home at least prevents them from drinking elsewhere and putting themselves at risk for other things. This is not entirely accurate, especially if there are no limits set on amount or frequency. Alcohol is damaging to the developing brain and can cause structural abnormalities as previously mentioned. You also increase the risk of a young child developing addictive behaviors.[12] Whether a few sips of alcohol as a teenager determines drinking behavior in the future is not necessarily pre-determined, but the more alcohol a young person drinks overtime the more exposure they have to its effects. Therefore, it is totally reasonable and responsible if you want to prevent exposure to alcohol for your children.

13. I just heard my daughter throwing up after dinner. I think she is purging her meals. How do I approach her about this?

Bulimia is a condition where someone has behaviors of bingeing and purging. It begins with some maladaptive cognitive beliefs about appearance. These individuals are usually unsatisfied with their body image and try to use purging to control the weight. Bulimia has significant deleterious medical consequences to the body. It can cause problems with dentition from the act of throwing up as well as the acidity of the vomit causing damage to teeth, corrosion of the esophagus, and it can cause an imbalance of electrolytes.[13] Individuals with Bulimia can develop skin infections from using their finger to purge, leaving open wounds that result from teeth marks that occur on fingers. In extreme cases it can affect the heart and can be fatal.[14]

Eating disorders require prompt attention. The first step would be making sure that you do not allow her to go to the bathroom immediately after eating, so that she is not able to throw up what she just ate. Monitoring her for about an hour after meals can help to set limits on purging. Also, she does require professional help for this. A doctor should order routine lab work to make sure her electrolytes and other metabolic functions are operating correctly. She needs a therapist to work with her on finding other ways to cope. There are intensive outpatient and inpatient programs when these behaviors continue and are deemed severe enough to require that level of attention.

The availability of resources to treat eating disorders poses a constant challenge to families who struggle with a child dealing with this. Now that telemedicine services are more routine due to the COVID-19 pandemic, some outpatient services can occur virtually. Find out if she has been bullied about her weight, and maybe encourage her to explore challenging her perceptions about body image. There may also need to be work done on the binge component of bulimia, such as working on appropriate portion sizes so that she does not feel as strong of an urge to then throw up. Eating disorders can be challenging to treat but there are also many success stories. Symptoms may flare at times of stress, but they can be managed with appropriate help.

14. If my teenage daughter shows interest in cooking and I teach her how, am I promoting gender roles? My husband does not cook at all, and it is only me making food for our family. Should my daughter grow up to just accept that? I do not want her to be taken for granted, with the same gender roles forced upon her.

Cooking can be fun it can be a bonding experience. You can even get a child interested in science, learning about the properties of different foods and how they interact with each other. I do not believe it should be discouraged if she has an interest in wanting to learn, it may be something she enjoys doing. It also fosters independence and pride in being able to create. You may have to teach her that even though it is not reflected at home, equal contribution in a partnership is important, and can include both partners contributing to cooking. I grew up in a home where my father also cooked so I grew up with that as part of my reality.

Many families have more traditional gender roles, many have role reversals. Your daughter will have to define her path going forward about what she is willing to contribute and what her expectations are from a partner. When people tell girls that they should learn to cook so that they can cook for their husbands, it is demeaning, can make them feel devalued, and cause your daughter to rebel, seeking a more non-traditional union intentionally. Putting women in a box and defining them by how well they do this is not helpful. Unfortunately, often the biggest critics and oppressors are other women such as critical and intrusive in-laws. You can encourage your child's interest in something like cooking that brings her joy, without propagating ideas around oppression.

15. My 18-year-old son is graduating from high school this year. He recently told me that he wants to be an actor. I told him that he should do that on the side while pursuing a more stable career path. I do not want to fund his college education if he does not take it seriously. Am I wrong in wanting security for him?

Do you remember all the dreams you had when you were young? I dreamed of being an astronaut, which I still daydream about sometimes. One exciting part of being young is having dreams and imagining them coming to fruition. If we did not have dreamers, we would not have astronauts, geologists, marine biologists, musicians, and inventors. Your concerns for your son are valid but I would not require him to dismiss his dreams. Perhaps you can discuss whether acting can be a minor area of study while he opts for another more "pragmatic" major as an option.

I have seen aspiring actors and models in a city like Los Angeles who face a lot of stress around paying bills when they do not have steady income. It can take a while to strike a balance between finding security and satisfying your passions. Many actors take jobs that provide them with the flexibility to go on auditions and take acting classes. A good friend of mine is an actor and a therapist. He has been able to pursue both. There are many people with dual careers, pursuing their passions of music, acting, comedy, art.

It is possible to pursue having career stability and a passion project, such as acting, which may not provide immediate or steady financial stability. It would be good for your son to meet other people who have found a way to nourish their acting passion and how they were able to do so. When I became involved with medical journalism, I met others who helped me create my path with having a creative outlet while practicing medicine.

Attending improvisation classes or acting workshops can help with public speaking and interviewing skills, and it builds confidence. You can be realistic and loving about your expectations while also being clear about what you are willing to do. If you decide that you can fund your son's college education if he agrees to also pursue a different opportunity while also pursuing acting, then have that conversation. One transition for a parent to make when their children become adults is accepting that the life your child chooses may not be exactly aligned with what you want and ultimately finding acceptance with their journey.

16. Should I get my teen a car? All her friends have one and she feels it is only fair she gets one.

With the advent of ridesharing, young people have alternatives to driving themselves places, although more recently due to COVID-19 there can be risks if appropriate public health measures are not followed. Many parents are also wary of allowing their teenagers to use ridesharing options especially being driven by people they do not know. Also, due to insurance costs many parents do not mind postponing their children getting behind the wheel. For others, allowing their teenager to drive gives them some freedom from having to schedule a time for drop-offs and pickups to various things. It is understandable to have anxiety about your child driving. Safety is also an important consideration.

You do not have to buy your daughter a car just because her friends have them. As a parent, you also do not have to succumb to peer pressure just to follow the same path as other parents around you. The decision to buy your child a vehicle is a decision made if it is right for your family both in a financial sense and taking into consideration whether your daughter can handle the responsibility of driving safely.

Before getting her a car, you should make sure she has some basic knowledge of different parts of the vehicle, how to handle emergencies, and how to drive in different weather conditions. If your teenager has a job, part of the financial budgeting may involve them having to contribute some of the money they make to car payments and/or insurance payments. It is more important that you are comfortable with this decision and can build a trusting relationship with your daughter to drive safely. Also, she must understand the importance of not driving under the influence of substances. Expose her to public service announcements and other content that discusses driver safety.

17. My 16-year-old son said he started to hear voices. What does this mean? His classmates do not understand what he is going through and tease him. How can I fight the stigma of mental illness and help him?

This is something that requires prompt medical attention, and he should be seen by a psychiatrist for further evaluation. Substances can cause symptoms of psychosis.[15][16] Teenagers can begin to experience hallucinations as a prodrome (early sign) to a psychotic mental illness.[17] They can also experience auditory and visual hallucinations if they were a victim of trauma, where they think they see or hear the perpetrator.[18]

Sometimes hallucinations can be mood congruent. This means when there is about of depression or mania (increased energy, elated or irritable mood, grandiose thinking, decreased need for sleep, increased goal-directed activity), an individual can experience hallucinations.[19] Early detection and intervention are important aspects of treatment.

It is important to create a nurturing, safe environment for your son to mitigate additional stress. You may have to explore educational options to minimize stress or have him take a leave of absence to focus on healing from mental illness. Parents sometimes want to share details with the school staff of their child's mental health issues with the hope that the school will accommodate and be more empathetic to their child. Others are worried about stigma so want to keep things private. It is also possible to let the school staff know your child is struggling and needs accommodations but without giving details. In the US, you can request an evaluation for an Individualized Education Plan that can serve to address specific issues your child deals with that can affect academic performance.

As far as teasing is concerned, the school staff should be vigilant about watching for signs of bullying and should intervene with consequences for those who engage in bullying. The school environment must be one where bullying is not tolerated. Sometimes the decision to change the academic environment is the best if it is one that does not seem supportive of the child's journey. In various parts of the world, there does not exist an understanding of mental health issues, people suffering from mental illness are shunned and ostracized. However, international mental health organizations are focusing on raising awareness and decreasing stigma around mental illness. The National Alliance on Mental Illness (NAMI) is one organization that provides informational materials about mental illness and provides support to family members that are dealing with a relative with mental illness. Finding out what resources are available locally and virtually can offer support in dealing with your child's mental health issues.

18. My daughter has scars on her arms from cutting herself. What do I do?

Self-injurious behaviors are concerning and can be a sign that your child is suffering from depression. Even though you may feel panic, approaching it from a calm angle of empathy may help her express to you why she did it. She may be experiencing bullying at school or feel stress from academic pressures. She may be dealing with depressive symptoms.[20] Sometimes people can cut simply to feel pain as a distraction from their emotional pain, sometimes it is a suicidal gesture. Self-injurious behaviors can occur when children have experienced trauma such as abuse.[21] This type of behavior is a sign to find her a therapist who is experienced with dealing with this.

Young people may cover their arms with long sleeves or other clothing to cover other parts of the body that they have cut, so it may not be clearly visible. It is important to know if your daughter is experiencing any thoughts of not wanting to be alive and request immediate help from a trained mental health professional if she is. A therapist can help your daughter learn different coping skills and a psychiatrist can evaluate to discern whether other types of treatment may be of benefit. When a child or teen displays self-injurious behaviors or uses items to try to harm others (or expresses thoughts about it), locking up knives and other sharp objects, cleaning substances, and pill bottles are recommended.

19. My 17-year-old son recently joined a band. They practice in our garage and are quite loud. I do not want to sabotage his dreams, but I feel like he is wasting his time. How do I handle this?

Musical expression can be uplifting for people. It also can build confidence grow as they become more comfortable over time with performing. Practicing music is a more positive activity than using drugs and alcohol (although some parents worry that their child's bandmates may be into both). There is perhaps a way that you can allow your child to experience the joy of making music but make it tolerable. One consideration is that loud music can be damaging to the ears and cause hearing loss. Educating him on that and requesting limits on noise pollution is important as it can protect against hearing loss. It may be safer for your child and his bandmates to wear earplugs if the music is loud. Also, you can set limits on when and how long they can practice in your garage, request for them to rotate locations where they practice, and at what volume you find acceptable. Talking to your child's pediatrician can help determine the safest way to engage in this activity while protecting his ears.

Learning an instrument can help with neural connectivity in the brain in a similar way that learning a language does.[22] If your son is expanding his musical skills, it can be a healthy process for your son's development. You can improve your ability to cope by perhaps taking a walk for a bit while they practice or wearing noise cancelling headphones. This may be a very cherished experience for your son and his friends, forming fond memories. Making music by itself does not have to be associated with other negative behaviors such as substance use. If you are suspicious that this may be an issue, you may want to come up with a plan that allows you appropriate supervision and giving your son some privacy to bond with his friends.

20. I am worried that my 19-year-old daughter is in an abusive relationship with a man 10 years older than her. He controls how much she communicates with her friends and family, how she spends her time, even what she wears. When she visits, he is constantly calling, wanting to know when she will be done. I have heard him yelling at her in a belittling way. One time I saw two fresh bruises on her arm, which she said she got from bumping into the door. How do I help her realize this relationship is not good for her?

Abuse is sadly all too common, and about one in four women in the US experience intimate partner violence according to the Centers for Disease Control and Prevention's (CDC) National Intimate Partner and Sexual Violence Survey (NISVS). You can start by checking in with your daughter on a regular basis, asking her if she is being treated all right. She may minimize the mistreatment. She may entertain beliefs that she is being treated this way because of something she did. She may feel confusion and feel disempowered in the relationship which affects her judgement.

Remind her that she deserves to be treated with respect and there are people, men included, who will do that. When we operate from a position of scarcity versus abundance, it may seem that this is all that is available to us, in terms of love. It is important to shift her perspective on this, but in such a way that she does not further shut down to avoid feeling judged. Leaving an abusive relationship can be difficult, partly due to feeling disempowered, and sometimes the abuse escalates when someone tries to leave. There is a risk of being seriously harmed or even killed when someone tries to leave an abusive situation, so this fear is justified.[23]

You can give her information about helpful resources that provide her with trained professionals she can speak with who understand her position. This may be more acceptable for your daughter, to speak with someone other than family and it can help guide her to make the right decision. Sometimes, a person does not realize that they are in an abusive relationship and she or he may not realize how bad it is. They will make excuses, get defensive, and support their abuser.

Many victims of abuse may claim that they instigated the abuser's anger. This shows the power of abuse, psychologically and physically. Even if the physical abuse stops, the emotional and psychological ramifications can continue. Steering away from patronizing advice that blames your daughter for not leaving or making better choices, but instead finding ways to empower her, will be more beneficial in the long run.

As a parent, it may be useful for you to contact a domestic violence support group or organization to find out how you can help your daughter. She can join many others who eventually get out of abusive relationships and begin the healing process. You may want your daughter to report to authorities about the abuse, but she may not want to disclose it. You can talk to law enforcement entities or domestic violence organizations to find out if there is something that can be done preemptively to prevent further violence. Intimate partner violence increases the risk of death by firearms.[24][25]

Sometimes, law enforcement can intervene early enough and prevent further violence. Due to reports of police brutality among people of color, many are hesitant to be involved with the police. There of course exists corruption within law enforcement agencies worldwide, and in many parts of the world still, a woman is blamed, even reprimanded if she reports abuse. Despite these unfortunate circumstances, having an external presence like law enforcement involved may be inevitable when there is abuse.

21. I found a pipe in my son's sock drawer, which he says belongs to a "friend." What is the appropriate way to deal with this?

The presence of drug paraphernalia should raise suspicion. You cannot prove that it is his friend's pipe, and you may not be able to prove that he is using drugs, but it should raise your level of caution with supervision. Curiosity about smoking cigarettes, drugs, and alcohol are common in adolescence, but not all young people act on it. You can decide to put in place consequences for possession of paraphernalia and be proactive about looking for it. You can randomly search his room but still allow your son some privacy for certain activities like writing in a journal. You must have a conversation about the deleterious effects of alcohol and drugs on the body and why it concerns you. You can decide on a plan about how your son can build your trust.

You do not want to constantly accuse him of using substances every time he does anything social because then it becomes a setup for him feeling he can never win your trust. It may also cause him to want to further rebel and it is not necessarily always productive. You want to have the parenting style of rewarding positive behaviors, even when there is history of rule infractions. It is also useful to monitor expendable cash your son has access to and consider getting outside help. There does exist a genetic component to substance dependence, and some young people are more prone to develop dependency as a result.[26] People can use substances to numb pain or escape from painful emotions and a therapist can help educate an individual on more positive ways of coping. Encouraging pro-social activities such as certain sports or clubs where he can associate with peers not using substances can help prevent the development of substance-related issues.

22. One of my friends said something quite unkind about my daughter. How do I talk to her about this?

People can say things that do not seem respectful based on their own emotions and if they are in a negative place. You can let her know that this hurt your feelings and it was extra painful to hear these things said about your daughter. Usually, when a person feels guilty about something they do, they are more likely to apologize. Others may feel shame about it and become defensive, making excuses for their behavior by justifying it.

Sometimes parents may feel jealous of another child's successes because they may be dealing with things related to their own children and families that they cannot control. As a result, they lash out at those who are close to them. Understanding that may not feel like much consolation but it can help you not take it personally.

Also, parents can be defensive about their own children's behavior, especially if it is the same type of behavior, they engage in. Not correcting the child who is engaging in disrespectful behavior is problematic and does not allow room for correction. Overly permissive attitudes with excessive praise without learning any consequences for negative behavior does not help a child treat others with compassion and empathy. A parent may become defensive when feedback is provided about their child even if it is warranted in the situation. Understanding where your friend is coming from and giving her a chance to explain or apologize can help you both work through this.

23. My daughter, who is 16, listens to disturbing music. Is this just a phase or does that mean she is exposing herself to negativity that will affect her later?

There are a lot of disturbing content themes in music out there.

Some young people listen to some of this content out of curiosity or simply enjoy the rhythm and melody. Sometimes the content is demeaning, focused on objectification, violence, and promiscuous sexual behavior. This can naturally be concerning to you. You do not want your daughter to believe that her worth is tied to her sexuality or that violence towards women or otherwise is permissible. You can have an open conversation with her about how you feel about it. Many young people will acknowledge that the much of the musical content is not that respectful of girls and women. They may also agree that there is a lot of aggressive language focused on violence in some music. It does not necessarily mean they will act out on those themes. Even students who excel and do not engage in problematic behavior can listen to music you find disturbing simply because it is catchy.

Young people may be interested in different kinds of much, they can appreciate classical music as well as rap music, for example. I was exposed to a lot of different kinds of music growing up and it has enriched my appreciation for different kinds of music. Many musical artists sing about drinking when they do not even drink alcohol because of a strict diet they are following. It becomes about an image rather than reflective of their lifestyle. It may be helpful for you and your daughter to understand some of these paradoxes concerning the marketing side of music. Music can also glorify what artists find pleasurable or highlight what they are struggling with themselves, such as addiction or dark moods. Amy Winehouse's deep, rich voice and soulful music often touched on painful emotions and hinted at her struggles with substances. Musicians who sing about material wealth may also be simultaneously dealing with financial problems that the listener is not aware of.

I do not suggest trying to quell your child's musical curiosity completely as they may just feel stifled. Instead having conversations about self-respect and the importance of what qualities we all possess on the inside can build your rapport. You can have an honest discussion explaining why you find some of the musical content troubling and your concerns about her having repeated exposure to it. She may eventually agree with you and not want to listen to the content you find disturbing. In some religious homes, children are not allowed to listen to any music that is not religious, and many of these children grow up to seek freedom concerning their auditory experiences. For example, Katy Perry has spoken about having restrictions around music growing up in a religious home as a child. Sometimes the experience can be positive being exposed to uplifting religious music, and sometimes it can also pique curiosity about other forms of music.

24. We live in an area where people are big on hunting, and my children want to try it, but I abhor guns and do not want my kids to go near them at all. How do I handle this?

Hunting is considered a sporting event by many people. Historically, people hunted to provide food for their families. Coming from a family of lifelong vegetarians, hunting is not something my family had any interest in ever. The violence of it is just not something I have been able to reconcile with. With climate change and research about meat causing cancer, adopting a more plant-based lifestyle is something that is recommended by many experts. You do not have to encourage hunting if it is against your value system or if you worry about safety. There are so many sporting events your children can be involved in that do not involve killing living things. It may be a much more valuable lesson that they learn empathy for other living things. Volunteering with conservation efforts may help them be close to nature in a kinder, more gentle way. Archery is a sport that may help with improving aim at a target without the violent aspect of hunting involved.

25. My 19-year-old Indian son recently told me that he is gay. He is struggling, feeling anxiety and sadness about not feeling accepted among his peers. My husband and I are okay with this and it will not change our relationship with him, but I am worried that people in our community will say hurtful things about him and to him. How do I protect him?

Congratulations on being open-minded and accepting of your son's experience. Coming out to family takes a lot of courage and is usually quite difficult to do. Many people feel like they are disappointing their parents for revealing this part of themselves. There are individuals who hold on to this secret throughout their life. In certain cultures, it is not widely accepted, which makes dealing with identity even more difficult. Hopefully, the dialogue and attitudes around homosexuality progress to a more accepting atmosphere worldwide. It is important to be supportive and accepting as a parent as your son can be dealing with his own fears and concerns about how he will be received to the world.

You want to make sure your son has access to information about safe sex practices, just as with any teenager, so he can make wise decisions. During this time, it can be useful to talk to a therapist. There are organizations that provide resources for the LGBTQ community, some specific to those of South Asian descent. You may not be control everything that is said in your community about you or your son. You can however allow your son his choice of how he wants to tell people or whether he even wants to bring it up with certain people. He can manage that on a need-to-know basis. Let him have the freedom to decide whom he would like to disclose this too and when he wants to share his story.

Do not tolerate disrespectful language about your son or homosexuality in your circles, and correct people when it happens. Calmly state your demand that he be treated with respect regardless of anyone's opinion about his sexual orientation. Homosexuality can be hard for many family members and others to accept across various cultures. They may worry your son will be victimized for his orientation, or they may have certain religious beliefs. You can discuss these things with family members and friends with your son's agreement as it pertains to him. You can explain to them that what he needs is support, not chastisement, ridicule, or judgment. You may have to set boundaries if the environment is not supportive. The more you can stand up for him, the more he will feel your love and feel confident to stand up for himself.

26. My daughter's father passed away before her 21st birthday and she was close to him. How do I help her manage her grief as well as mine?

Loss is an inevitable part of life. In the west, we often try our best to shield ourselves from it, and we have an expectation to live long, productive lives. There are different types of loss, loss of a parent, loss of a relationship, loss of a child, loss of livelihood. If we change our perspective about loss, sometimes it can be a profound growth experience.

I often recommend the book "Life after Loss" by Bob Deits to patients and friends. Deits worked as a pastor who would support parents who were dealing with their babies breathing their final moments. Deits talks about grief as a continuum that you create a manageable relationship, as opposed to something to immediately overcome.

"There is no quota system to the number of losses we can experience in life. Learning how to cope with our losses and regain a sense of "normal" is one of the most important skills any of us can develop. Even when we are not experiencing a major loss ourselves, we know others who are, and we wonder what we can say or do." Bob Deits

Loss makes us human, it unifies, divides, builds and breaks bridges. It can test our system, our stress responses, illustrate the capacity for love. Often the pain feels excruciating, like there will be no escape from it. I once saw a child patient whose younger brother was killed after being hit by a vehicle. Her mother committed suicide a year later and she was in the custody of a maternal cousin. The mother could not reconcile with the pain of losing her child. Her surviving family members, including her young daughter had over time developed a sanguine understanding and sympathy for what mom had endured. They did not focus on the abandonment of the other living child, or bare anger towards mom for doing what she did.

Could this mother have explored different options after being confronted with this terrible loss? Could she have, not despite her pain, but because of it, turn her attention towards an alternative purpose? We all handle loss at different frequencies and healing trajectories. One may wonder how the future of her surviving child differ if her mother could channel her grief towards supporting her living child's journey? When you are under the fog of enormous grief, it can be nearly impossible to see any other alternative of being, and in this case, the only viable option seemed to be leaving this life. However, those alternative choices maybe critical in making life choices affecting you and your family members.

I once met a mother who lost two of her sons, one in an accident and one from an overdose attempt. She had custody of her grandchildren. She told me it kept her going because there was no other choice. I have been affected by suicide of two friends. I had spoken to one a few days prior and did not realize she was contemplating ending her life. To this day I sometimes wonder if something could have been done to prevent the loss of my friends. Questions like this often plague our minds when dealing with loss. The method of inquiry, "Who Am I?" can be useful in times of loss. You are someone's daughter or son, someone's mother or father, someone's friend, lover, confidant, neighbor. You are needed and valuable.

> "Something very beautiful happens to people when their world has fallen apart: a humility, a nobility, a higher intelligence emerges at just the point when our knees hit the floor. Perhaps, in a way, that's where humanity is now: about to discover we are not as smart as we thought we were, will be forced by life to surrender our attacks and defenses which avail us of nothing, and finally break through into the collective beauty of who we really are."
>
> --Marianne Williamson

Instead of fearing the inevitability of loss, we would be better served understanding the process and appreciating what factors we can and cannot control. People who exhibit resilience in the face of adversity tend to do better in terms of overall health and wellbeing. Holocaust survivors, those who have overcome famine, war, and made something out of the experience demonstrated the quality of resilience. This is not a character asset that necessarily comes from an education, it is something that can be developed. Humans by nature are a resilient species and have learned to adapt and reinvent themselves throughout time. If, like Deits tells us, we could strengthen our resilience, it may help us to cope, cherish moments of joy, feel interconnected, and not alone.

CONCLUSION

These questions and answers give just a brief glimpse of the various topics that parents have brought to my attention. It has been a privilege to watch how love for a child can encourage parents to work on the flexibility of the mind, show a willingness to grow and change, and how they can work on themselves. There are no quick and easy answers to what ensures a well-adjusted adult, it is a complicated interplay between genetics, environment, life experiences, and psychological temperament that shapes our resilience. However, an attitude of compassion, empathy, and acceptance can be transformative for a child. Not projecting your issues onto your child can be a difficult balancing act, and an uphill battle, but one that is worth fighting for. I have seen the damage narcissism, abuse, and other trauma can have on a child, affecting mental and physical health. There does always exist opportunities to repair, build self-esteem, cultivate values of compassion and empathy, while instilling many moments of unbridled joy that every child deserves to experience. It is the small steps of your personal growth as a parent, uncle, or aunt, grandparent, teacher, or mentor to a child that matter, you would be surprised at how powerful some of the smallest actions can be.

"History will judge us by the difference we make in the everyday lives of children."

--Nelson Mandela

REFERENCES

THE EARLY YEARS

1. Thompson, R. A. (1998). Early sociopersonality development.
2. Denham, S. (1998). Emotional Development in Young Children. New York: Guilford.
3. Fogel, A. (1993). Developing Through Relationships: Origins of communication, self, and culture. Chicago: University of Chicago Press.
4. Shonkoff, J.P., & Phillips, D. (Eds.) (2000). From Neurons to Neighborhoods: The science of early childhood development. Committee on Integrating the Science of Early Childhood Development. Washington, DC: National Academy Press.
5. Lavelli, M., & Fogel, A. (2005). Developmental changes in the relationship between the infant's attention and emotion during early face-to-face communication: the 2-month transition. Developmental psychology, 41(1), 265.
6. Braungart-Rieker, J. M., Hill-Soderlund, A. L., &Karrass, J. (2010). Fear and anger reactivity trajectories from 4 to 16 months: The roles of temperament, regulation, and maternal sensitivity. Developmental psychology, 46(4), 791.
7. LeDoux, J. (2000). Emotion circuits in the brain. Annual Review of Neuroscience, 23, 155-184.
8. Saarni, C., Campos, J. J., Camras, L. A., & Witherington, D. (2007). Emotional development: Action, communication, and understanding. Handbook of child psychology, 3.
9. Brooker, R. J., Buss, K. A., Lemery-Chalfant, K., Aksan, N., Davidson, R. J., & Goldsmith, H. H. (2013). The development of stranger fear in infancy and toddlerhood: normative development, individual differences, antecedents, and outcomes. Developmental science, 16(6), 864-878.
10. Brand, R. J., Escobar, K., & Patrick, A. M. (2020). Coincidence or cascade? The temporal relation between locomotor behaviors and the emergence of stranger anxiety. Infant Behavior and Development, 58, 101423.
11. Williams, J. H., Waiter, G. D., Perra, O., Perrett, D. I., & Whiten, A. (2005). An fMRI study of joint attention experience. Neuroimage, 25(1), 133-140.
12. Saunders, T. J., & Vallance, J. K. (2017). Screen time and health indicators among children and youth: current evidence, limitations and future directions. Applied health economics and health policy, 15(3), 323-331.
13. Thomas, R., Sanders, S., Doust, J., Beller, E., & Glasziou, P. (2015). Prevalence of attention-deficit/hyperactivity disorder: a systematic review and meta-analysis. Pediatrics, 135(4), e994-e1001.
14. Becker, S. P. (2020). ADHD and sleep: recent advances and future directions. Current opinion in psychology, 34, 50-56.

15. Stringham, J. M., Johnson, E. J., & Hammond, B. R. (2019). Lutein across the lifespan: from childhood cognitive performance to the aging eye and brain. *Current developments in nutrition*, 3(7), nzz066.
16. Rohlfs Domínguez P. (2020). New insights into the ontogeny of human vegetable consumption: From developmental brain and cognitive changes to behavior. *Developmental cognitive neuroscience*, 45, 100830. https://doi.org/10.1016/j.dcn.2020.100830
17. Grantham-McGregor, S., & Smith, J. (2020). The Effect of Malnutrition and Micronutrient Deficiency on Children's Mental Health. *Mental Health and Illness of Children and Adolescents*, 375-393.
18. Effatpanah, M., Rezaei, M., Effatpanah, H., Effatpanah, Z., Varkaneh, H. K., Mousavi, S. M., ... & Hashemi, R. (2019). Magnesium status and attention deficit hyperactivity disorder (ADHD): A meta-analysis. *Psychiatry research*, 274, 228-234.
19. Derbyshire, E. (2017). Do omega-3/6 fatty acids have a therapeutic role in children and young people with ADHD?. *Journal of lipids*, 2017.
20. Esposito, S., Laino, D., D'Alonzo, R., Mencarelli, A., Di Genova, L., Fattorusso, A., ... & Mencaroni, E. (2019). Pediatric sleep disturbances and treatment with melatonin. *Journal of translational medicine*, 17(1), 1-8.
21. Rehm, J., Gmel Sr, G. E., Gmel, G., Hasan, O. S., Imtiaz, S., Popova, S., ... & Shuper, P. A. (2017). The relationship between different dimensions of alcohol use and the burden of disease—an update. *Addiction*, 112(6), 968-1001.
22. Bagge, C. L., & Borges, G. (2017). Acute substance use as a warning sign for suicide attempts: a case-crossover examination of the 48 hours prior to a recent suicide attempt. *The Journal of clinical psychiatry*, 78(6), 691-696.
23. Møller, A. P., & Cuervo, J. J. (2000). The evolution of paternity and paternal care in birds. *Behavioral* Ecology, 11(5), 472-485.
24. Gopurenko, D., Williams, R. N., McCormick, C. R., & DeWOODY, J. A. (2006). Insights into the mating habits of the tiger salamander (Ambystoma tigrinum tigrinum) as revealed by genetic parentage analyses. *Molecular Ecology*, 15(7), 1917-1928.
25. DeWoody, J. A., & Avise, J. C. (2001). Genetic perspectives on the natural history of fish mating systems. *Journal of Heredity*, 92(2), 167-172.
26. Brooker, R. J., Buss, K. A., Lemery-Chalfant, K., Aksan, N., Davidson, R. J., & Goldsmith, H. H. (2013). The development of stranger fear in infancy and toddlerhood: normative development, individual differences, antecedents, and outcomes. *Developmental science*, 16(6), 864-878.
27. Schulz, R., & Sherwood, P. R. (2008). Physical and mental health effects of family caregiving. *Journal of Social Work Education*, 44(sup3), 105-113..
28. Fullerton, J. M., Totsika, V., Hain, R., & Hastings, R. P. (2017). Siblings of children with life-limiting conditions: Psychological adjustment and sibling relationships. *Child: care, health and development*, 43(3), 393-400.
29. Deavin, A., Greasley, P., & Dixon, C. (2018). Children's perspectives on living with a sibling with a chronic illness. *Pediatrics*, 142(2).
30. Horne, Z., Powell, D., Hummel, J. E., & Holyoak, K. J. (2015). Countering anti-vaccination attitudes. *Proceedings of the National Academy of Sciences*, 112(33), 10321-10324.
31. Shams-White, M. M., Brockton, N. T., Mitrou, P., Romaguera, D., Brown, S., Bender, A., ... & Reedy, J. (2019). Operationalizing the 2018 World Cancer

Research Fund/American Institute for Cancer Research (WCRF/AICR) cancer prevention recommendations: a standardized scoring system. *Nutrients*, 11(7), 1572.
32. Rock, C. L., Thomson, C., Gansler, T., Gapstur, S. M., McCullough, M. L., Patel, A. V., ... & Doyle, C. (2020). American Cancer Society guideline for diet and physical activity for cancer prevention. *CA: a cancer journal for clinicians*, 70(4), 245-271.
33. Zeraatkar, D., Han, M. A., Guyatt, G. H., Vernooij, R. W., El Dib, R., Cheung, K., ... & Johnston, B. C. (2019). Red and processed meat consumption and risk for all-cause mortality and cardiometabolic outcomes: a systematic review and meta-analysis of cohort studies. *Annals of internal medicine*, 171(10), 703-710.
34. Van Horn, N. L., & Street, M. (2018). Night Terrors.
35. Etain, B., Lajnef, M., Bellivier, F., Mathieu, F., Raust, A., Cochet, B., ... & Elgrabli, O. (2012). Clinical expression of bipolar disorder type I as a function of age and polarity at onset: convergent findings in samples from France and the United States. *The Journal of clinical psychiatry*, 73(4), 561-566.
36. Perlis, R. H., Miyahara, S., Marangell, L. B., Wisniewski, S. R., Ostacher, M., DelBello, M. P., ... & STEP-BD Investigators. (2004). Long-term implications of early onset in bipolar disorder: data from the first 1000 participants in the systematic treatment enhancement program for bipolar disorder (STEP-BD). *Biological psychiatry*, 55(9), 875-881.
37. Post, R. M., Altshuler, L. L., Kupka, R., McElroy, S. L., Frye, M. A., Rowe, M., ... & Nolen, W. A. (2017). More childhood onset bipolar disorder in the United States than Canada or Europe: Implications for treatment and prevention. *Neuroscience & Biobehavioral Reviews*, 74, 204-213.
38. Axelson, D., Goldstein, B., Goldstein, T., Monk, K., Yu, H., Hickey, M. B., ... & Birmaher, B. (2015). Diagnostic precursors to bipolar disorder in offspring of parents with bipolar disorder: a longitudinal study. *American Journal of Psychiatry*, 172(7), 638-646.
39. Saudino, K. J. (2005). Behavioral genetics and child temperament. *Journal of developmental and behavioral pediatrics: JDBP*, 26(3), 214.
40. Stringaris, A., Maughan, B., Copeland, W. S., Costello, E. J., & Angold, A. (2013). Irritable mood as a symptom of depression in youth: prevalence, developmental, and clinical correlates in the Great Smoky Mountains Study. *Journal of the American Academy of Child & Adolescent Psychiatry*, 52(8), 831-840.
41. Aas, M., Henry, C., Andreassen, O. A., Bellivier, F., Melle, I., & Etain, B. (2016). The role of childhood trauma in bipolar disorders. *International journal of bipolar disorders*, 4(1), 1-10.
42. Post, R. M., Altshuler, L. L., Kupka, R., McElroy, S. L., Frye, M. A., Rowe, M., ... & Nolen, W. A. (2015). Verbal abuse, like physical and sexual abuse, in childhood is associated with an earlier onset and more difficult course of bipolar disorder. *Bipolar disorders*, 17(3), 323-330.
43. Miklowitz, D. J., & Chung, B. (2016). Family-focused therapy for bipolar disorder: Reflections on 30 years of research. *Family process*, 55(3), 483-499.
44. McNamara, R. K., Nandagopal, J. J., Strakowski, S. M., & DelBello, M. P. (2010). Preventative strategies for early-onset bipolar disorder. *CNS drugs*, 24(12), 983-996.

45. Cotton, S., Kraemer, K. M., Sears, R. W., Strawn, J. R., Wasson, R. S., McCune, N., ... & Delbello, M. P. (2020). Mindfulness-based cognitive therapy for children and adolescents with anxiety disorders at-risk for bipolar disorder: A psychoeducation waitlist controlled pilot trial. *Early intervention in psychiatry*, 14(2), 211-219.
46. Hudziak, J. J., Albaugh, M. D., Ducharme, S., Karama, S., Spottswood, M., Crehan, E., ... & Brain Development Cooperative Group. (2014). Cortical thickness maturation and duration of music training: health-promoting activities shape brain development. *Journal of the American Academy of Child & Adolescent Psychiatry*, 53(11), 1153-1161.
47. Otto, M. W., Henin, A., Hirshfeld-Becker, D. R., Pollack, M. H., Biederman, J., & Rosenbaum, J. F. (2007). Posttraumatic stress disorder symptoms following media exposure to tragic events: Impact of 9/11 on children at risk for anxiety disorders. *Journal of anxiety disorders*, 21(7), 888-902.
48. Staggers-Hakim, R. (2016). The nation's unprotected children and the ghost of Mike Brown, or the impact of national police killings on the health and social development of African American boys. *Journal of Human Behavior in the Social Environment*, **26**(3-4), 390–399.
49. Funk, J. B., Baldacci, H. B., Pasold, T., & Baumgardner, J. (2004). Violence exposure in real-life, video games, television, movies, and the internet: is there desensitization?. *Journal of adolescence*, 27(1), 23-39.
50. Thomas, M. H., Horton, R. W., Lippincott, E. C., & Drabman, R. S. (1977). Desensitization to portrayals of real-life aggression as a function of television violence. *Journal of personality and social psychology*, 35(6), 450.
51. Chapman, D. P., Whitfield, C. L., Felitti, V. J., Dube, S. R., Edwards, V. J., & Anda, R. F. (2004). Adverse childhood experiences and the risk of depressive disorders in adulthood. *Journal of affective disorders*, 82(2), 217-225.

CHILDHOOD

1. Schieltz, K. M., Wacker, D. P., & Romani, P. W. (2017). Effects of signaled positive reinforcement on problem behavior maintained by negative reinforcement. *Journal of Behavioral Education*, 26(2), 137-150.
2. Iverach, L., Jones, M., McLellan, L. F., Lyneham, H. J., Menzies, R. G., Onslow, M., &Rapee, R. M. (2016). Prevalence of anxiety disorders among children who stutter. *Journal of Fluency Disorders*, 49, 13-28.
3. Hosseinkhanzadeh, A. A., Shakerinia, I., &Baradran, M. (2016). Effectiveness of Assertiveness Skills Training on Decreasing Social Anxiety of Children with Stuttering. *Middle Eastern Journal of Disability Studies*, 6, 164-170.
4. Guerra, M. R. V., Estelles, J. R. D., Abdouni, Y. A., Falcochio, D. F., Rosa, J. R. P., & Catani, L. H. (2016). Frequency of wrist growth plate injury in young gymnasts at a training center. *Acta ortopedica brasileira*, 24(4), 204-207.
5. Saluan, P., Styron, J., Ackley, J. F., Prinzbach, A., & Billow, D. (2015). Injury types and incidence rates in precollegiate female gymnasts: a 21-year experience at a single training facility. *Orthopaedic journal of sports medicine*, 3(4), 2325967115577596.

REFERENCES | 173

6. Hammer, A., Schwartzbach, A. L., & Paulev, P. E. (1981). Trampoline training injuries--one hundred and ninety-five cases. *British journal of sports medicine*, 15(3), 151-158.
7. Mohriak, R., Silva, P. D. V., Trandafilov Jr, M., Martins, D. E., Wajchenberg, M., Cohen, M., & Puertas, E. B. (2010). Spondylolysis and spondylolisthesis in young gymnasts. *Revista Brasileira de Ortopedia (English Edition)*, 45(1), 79-83.
8. Kolt, G. S., & Kirkby, R. J. (1999). Epidemiology of injury in elite and subelite female gymnasts: a comparison of retrospective and prospective findings. *British journal of sports medicine*, 33(5), 312-318.
9. Hart, E., Meehan III, W. P., Bae, D. S., d'Hemecourt, P., & Stracciolini, A. (2018). The young injured gymnast: a literature review and discussion. *Current sports medicine reports*, 17(11), 366-375.
10. Rex, M. A. (2018). Racial Bias in Elementary School Children: Effects of Skin Tone and Facial Features.
11. Bryant-Davis, T., & Ocampo, C. (2006). A therapeutic approach to the treatment of racist-incident-based trauma. *Journal of Emotional Abuse*, 6(4), 1-22.
12. Comas-Díaz, L. (2016). Racial trauma recovery: A race-informed therapeutic approach to racial wounds. In Alvarez, A.N. (Ed); Liang, C. T. H. (Ed); Neville, H. A. (Ed), The cost of racism for people of color: Contextualizing experiences of discrimination. Cultural, racial, and ethnic psychology book series (pp. 249-272). Washington, DC, US: American Psychological Association.
13. Jones, S. C., Anderson, R. E., Gaskin-Wasson, A. L., Sawyer, B. A., Applewhite, K., & Metzger, I. W. (2020). From "crib to coffin": Navigating coping from racism-related stress throughout the lifespan of Black Americans. *American Journal of Orthopsychiatry*, 90(2), 267.
14. Paradies, Y., Ben, J., Denson, N., Elias, A., Priest, N., Pieterse, A., ... & Gee, G. (2015). Racism as a determinant of health: a systematic review and meta-analysis. *PloS one*, 10(9), e0138511.
15. Tangel, V., White, R. S., Nachamie, A. S., & Pick, J. S. (2019). Racial and ethnic disparities in maternal outcomes and the disadvantage of peripartum black women: a multistate analysis, 2007–2014. *American journal of perinatology*, 36(08), 835-848.
16. Bougie, O., Healey, J., & Singh, S. S. (2019). Behind the times: revisiting endometriosis and race. *American journal of obstetrics and gynecology*, 221(1), 35-e1.
17. Taran, F. A., Brown, H. L., & Stewart, E. A. (2010). Racial diversity in uterine leiomyoma clinical studies. Fertility and sterility, 94(4), 1500-1503.
18. Collins, F. S., Morgan, M., &Patrinos, A. (2003). The Human Genome Project: lessons from large-scale biology. *Science*, 300(5617), 286-290.
19. Mitchell, M. M., Armstrong, G., & Armstrong, T. (2020). Disproportionate school disciplinary responses: An exploration of prisonization and minority threat hypothesis among black, Hispanic, and Native American students. *Criminal Justice Policy Review*, 31(1), 80-102.
20. Owens, J., & McLanahan, S. S. (2020). Unpacking the drivers of racial disparities in school suspension and expulsion. *Social Forces*, 98(4), 1548-1577.
21. Pachter, L. M., & Coll, C. G. (2009). Racism and child health: a review of the literature and future directions. *Journal of developmental and behavioral pediatrics: JDBP*, 30(3), 255.

22. Nyborg, V. M., & Curry, J. F. (2003). The impact of perceived racism: Psychological symptoms among African American boys. *Journal of Clinical Child and Adolescent Psychology*, 32(2), 258-266.
23. Cassiers, L. L., Sabbe, B. G., Schmaal, L., Veltman, D. J., Penninx, B. W., & Van Den Eede, F. (2018). Structural and functional brain abnormalities associated with exposure to different childhood trauma subtypes: A systematic review of neuroimaging findings. *Frontiers in psychiatry*, 9, 329.
24. Teicher, M. H. (2018). Childhood trauma and the enduring consequences of forcibly separating children from parents at the United States border. *BMC medicine*, 16(1), 1-3.
25. Taylor, C. (2021). *Fight the Power: African Americans and the Long History of Police Brutality in New York City*. NYU Press.
26. Ruch, D. A., Sheftall, A. H., Schlagbaum, P., Rausch, J., Campo, J. V., & Bridge, J. A. (2019). Trends in suicide among youth aged 10 to 19 years in the United States, 1975 to 2016. *JAMA network open*, 2(5), e193886-e193886.
27. Wang, P. W., & Yen, C. F. (2017). Adolescent substance use behavior and suicidal behavior for boys and girls: a cross-sectional study by latent analysis approach. *BMC psychiatry*, 17(1), 1-7.
28. Simmonds, M., Llewellyn, A., Owen, C. G., &Woolacott, N. (2016). Predicting adult obesity from childhood obesity: a systematic review and meta-analysis. *Obesity reviews*, 17(2), 95-107.
29. Fuemmeler, B. F., Lovelady, C. A., Zucker, N. L., &Østbye, T. (2013). Parental obesity moderates the relationship between childhood appetitive traits and weight. *Obesity (Silver Spring, Md.)*, 21(4), 815–823. https://doi.org/10.1002/oby.20144
30. Lifshitz F. (2008). Obesity in children. *Journal of clinical research in pediatric endocrinology*, 1(2), 53–60. https://doi.org/10.4008/jcrpe.v1i2.35
31. Sahoo, K., Sahoo, B., Choudhury, A. K., Sofi, N. Y., Kumar, R., & Bhadoria, A. S. (2015). Childhood obesity: causes and consequences. *Journal of family medicine and primary care*, 4(2), 187.
32. Skinner, AC, Steiner, MJ, Henderson, FW, Perrin, EM. Multiple markers of inflammation and weight status: cross-sectional analyses throughout childhood. Pediatrics. 2010;125:e801-e809.
33. Lakshman, R., Elks, C. E., & Ong, K. K. (2012). Childhood obesity. *Circulation*, 126(14), 1770-1779.
34. Staniford, L. J., Breckon, J. D., & Copeland, R. J. (2012). Treatment of childhood obesity: A systematic review. *Journal of Child and Family Studies*, 21(4), 545-564..
35. Raudsepp, L., &Kais, K. (2019). Longitudinal associations between problematic social media use and depressive symptoms in adolescent girls. *Preventive medicine reports*, 15, 100925.

ADOLESCENCE

1. Correll, J., &Keesee, T. (2009). Racial bias in the decision to shoot. *The Police Chief*, 76(5), 54-57.
2. Correll, J., Park, B., Judd, C. M., Wittenbrink, B., Sadler, M. S., &Keesee, T. (2007). Across the thin blue line: police officers and racial bias in the decision to

shoot. *Journal of personality and social psychology, 92*(6), 1006.
3. Eberhardt, J. L., Davies, P. G., Purdie-Vaughns, V. J., & Johnson, S. L. (2006). Looking death worthy: Perceived stereotypicality of Black defendants predicts capital-sentencing outcomes. *Psychological science, 17*(5), 383-386.
4. Jones, J. M., & Bryant-Davis, T. (2013). Race always matters. *Diversity US*.
5. Goff, P. A., Jackson, M. C., Di Leone, B. A. L., Culotta, C. M., & DiTomasso, N. A. (2014). The essence of innocence: consequences of dehumanizing Black children. *Journal of personality and social psychology, 106*(4), 526.
6. Pachter, L. M., & Coll, C. G. (2009). Racism and child health: a review of the literature and future directions. *Journal of developmental and behavioral pediatrics: JDBP, 30*(3), 255.
7. Jaffe, A. E., DiLillo, D., Gratz, K. L., & Messman-Moore, T. L. (2019). Risk for revictimization following interpersonal and noninterpersonal trauma: Clarifying the role of posttraumatic stress symptoms and trauma-related cognitions. *Journal of traumatic stress, 32*(1), 42-55.
8. Gould, M. S., Lake, A. M., Kleinman, M., Galfalvy, H., Chowdhury, S., & Madnick, A. (2018). Exposure to suicide in high schools: Impact on serious suicidal ideation/behavior, depression, maladaptive coping strategies, and attitudes toward help-seeking. *International journal of environmental research and public health, 15*(3), 455.
9. Lee, J. B., Affeldt, B. M., Gamboa, Y., Hamer, M., Dunn, J. F., Pardo, A. C., & Obenaus, A. (2018). Repeated pediatric concussions evoke long-term oligodendrocyte and white matter microstructural dysregulation distant from the injury. *Developmental neuroscience, 40*(4), 358-375.
10. Moksnes, U. K., & Espnes, G. A. (2013). Self-esteem and life satisfaction in adolescents—gender and age as potential moderators. *Quality of Life Research, 22*(10), 2921-2928.
11. Moksnes, U. K., &Espnes, G. A. (2012). Self-esteem and emotional health in adolescents–gender and age as potential moderators. *Scandinavian Journal of Psychology, 53*(6), 483-489.
12. Erol, R. Y., & Orth, U. (2011). Self-esteem development from age 14 to 30 years: A longitudinal study. *Journal of personality and social psychology, 101*(3), 607.
13. Andersen, S., Ertac, S., Gneezy, U., List, J. A., & Maximiano, S. (2013). Gender, competitiveness, and socialization at a young age: Evidence from a matrilineal and a patriarchal society. *Review of Economics and Statistics, 95*(4), 1438-1443.
14. Buser, T., Peter, N., & Wolter, S. C. (2017). Gender, willingness to compete and career choices along the whole ability distribution.
15. Graf, N., Brown, A., & Patten, E. (2018). The narrowing, but persistent, gender gap in pay. *Pew Research Center, 9*.
16. Bianchi, S. M., Milkie, M. A., Sayer, L. C., & Robinson, J. P. (2000). Is anyone doing the housework? Trends in the gender division of household labor. *Social forces, 79*(1), 191-228.
17. Campbell, J. C., Webster, D., Koziol-McLain, J., Block, C., Campbell, D., Curry, M. A., Gary, F., Glass, N., McFarlane, J., Sachs, C., Sharps, P., Ulrich, Y., Wilt, S. A., Manganello, J., Xu, X., Schollenberger, J., Frye, V., & Laughon, K. (2003). Risk factors for femicide in abusive relationships: results from a multisite case control study. *American journal of public health, 93*(7), 1089–1097. https://doi.org/10.2105/ajph.93.7.1089

REFERENCES

18. Jacobus, J., & Tapert, S. F. (2014). Effects of cannabis on the adolescent brain. *Current pharmaceutical design*, 20(13), 2186–2193. https://doi.org/10.2174/1381612811319999042 6
19. Raudsepp, L., &Kais, K. (2019). Longitudinal associations between problematic social media use and depressive symptoms in adolescent girls. *Preventive medicine reports*, 15, 100925.
20. Ortiz, R., & Sibinga, E. M. (2017). The role of mindfulness in reducing the adverse effects of childhood stress and trauma. *Children*, 4(3), 16.
21. Golland, Y., Golland, P., Bentin, S., &Malach, R. (2008). Data-driven clustering reveals a fundamental subdivision of the human cortex into two global systems. *Neuropsychologia*, 46(2), 540-553.
22. Gusnard, D. A., and Raichle, M. E. (2001). Searching for a baseline: functional imaging and the resting human brain. *Nat. Rev. Neurosci.* 2, 685–694.
23. Fransson, P. (2006). How default is the default mode of brain function? Further evidence from intrinsic BOLD signal fluctuations. *Neuropsychologia* 44, 2836–2845.
24. Fox, M. D., and Raichle, M. E. (2007). Spontaneous fluctuations in brain activity observed with functional magnetic resonance imaging. *Nat. Rev. Neurosci.* 8, 700–711.
25. Golland, Y., Bentin, S., Gelbard, H., Benjamini, Y., Heller, R., Nir, Y., Hasson, U., and Malach, R. (2007). Extrinsic and intrinsic systems in the posterior cortex of the human brain revealed during natural sensory stimulation. *Cereb. Cortex* 4, 766–777.
26. Golland, Y., Golland, P., Bentin, S., and Malach, R. (2008). Data-driven clustering reveals a fundamental subdivision of the human cortex into two global systems. *Neuropsychologia* 46, 540–553.
27. Tian, L., Jiang, T., Liu, Y., Yu, C., Wang, K., Zhou, Y., Song, M., and Li, K. (2007). The relationship within and between the extrinsic and intrinsic systems indicated by resting state correlational patterns of sensory cortices. *Neuroimage* 36, 684–69
28. Fox, M. D., Snyder, A. Z., Vincent, J. L., Corbetta, M., Van Essen, D. C., &Raichle, M. E. (2005). The human brain is intrinsically organized into dynamic, anticorrelated functional networks. *Proceedings of the National Academy of Sciences*, 102(27), 9673-9678.
29. Mennes, M., Zuo, X. N., Kelly, C., Di Martino, A., Zang, Y. F., Biswal, B., ... &Milham, M. P. (2011). Linking inter-individual differences in neural activation and behavior to intrinsic brain dynamics. *Neuroimage*, 54(4), 2950-2959.
30. Gusnard, D. A., and Raichle, M. E. (2001). Searching for a baseline: functional imaging and the resting human brain. *Nat. Rev. Neurosci.* 2, 685–694.
31. Fox, M. D., Snyder, A. Z., Vincent, J. L., Corbetta, M., Van Essen, D. C., & Raichle, M. E. (2005). The human brain is intrinsically organized into dynamic, anticorrelated functional networks. *Proceedings of the National Academy of Sciences*, 102(27), 9673-9678.
32. Josipovic, Z., Dinstein, I., Weber, J., &Heeger, D. J. (2012). Influence of meditation on anti-correlated networks in the brain. *Frontiers in human neuroscience*, 5, 183.
33. Josipovic, Z. (2014). Neural correlates of nondual awareness in meditation. *Annals of the New York Academy of Sciences*, 1307(1), 9-18.

34. Beck, A. T. (1993). Cognitive therapy: Past, present, and future. *Journal of Consulting and Clinical Psychology*, 61(2), 194-198. https://doi.org/10.1037/0022-006X.61.2.194
35. Hollon, S. D., & Beck, A. T. (2013). Cognitive and cognitive-behavioral therapies. *Bergin and Garfield's handbook of psychotherapy and behavior change*, 6, 393-442.
36. Hollon, et al., (2013)
37. Han, D. H., Lee, Y. S., Yang, K. C., Kim, E. Y., Lyoo, I. K., & Renshaw, P. F. (2007). Dopamine genes and reward dependence in adolescents with excessive internet video game play. *Journal of addiction medicine*, 1(3), 133-138.
38. Koepp, M. J., Gunn, R. N., Lawrence, A. D., Cunningham, V. J., Dagher, A., Jones, T., ... &Grasby, P. M. (1998). Evidence for striatal dopamine release during a video game. *Nature*, 393(6682), 266-268.
39. Kuss, D. J., & Griffiths, M. D. (2012). Internet and gaming addiction: a systematic literature review of neuroimaging studies. *Brain sciences*, 2(3), 347-374.
40. Volkow, N. D., Wang, G. J., Telang, F., Fowler, J. S., Logan, J., Childress, A. R., ... & Wong, C. (2006). Cocaine cues and dopamine in dorsal striatum: mechanism of craving in cocaine addiction. *Journal of Neuroscience*, 26(24), 6583-6588.
41. Koulouris, S., Pastromas, S., Sakellariou, D., Kratimenos, T., Piperopoulos, P., & Manolis, A. S. (2010). Takotsubo cardiomyopathy: the "broken heart" syndrome. *Hellenic J Cardiol*, 51(5), 451-7.
42. Baumeister, R. F., Wotman, S. R., & Stillwell, A. M. (1993). Unrequited love: On heartbreak, anger, guilt, scriptlessness, and humiliation. *Journal of Personality and Social Psychology*, 64(3), 377.
43. Baumeister, et al., (1993)
44. Baumeister, et al., (1993)
45. Fisher, H., Aron, A., & Brown, L. L. (2005). Romantic love: an fMRI study of a neural mechanism for mate choice. *Journal of Comparative Neurology*, 493(1), 58-62.
46. Earp, B. D., Wudarczyk, O. A., Foddy, B., & Savulescu, J. (2017). Addicted to love: What is love addiction and when should it be treated?. *Philosophy, psychiatry, &psychology : PPP*, 24(1), 77–92. https://doi.org/10.1353/ppp.2017.0011
47. Harden, K. P., & Tucker-Drob, E. M. (2011). Individual differences in the development of sensation seeking and impulsivity during adolescence: further evidence for a dual systems model. *Developmental psychology*, 47(3), 739.
48. Romer, D. (2010). Adolescent risk taking, impulsivity, and brain development: Implications for prevention. *Developmental Psychobiology: The Journal of the International Society for Developmental Psychobiology*, 52(3), 263-276.
49. Fisher, H. E., Aron, A., & Mashek, D. Haifang Li, and Lucy L. Brown. 2002.". *Defining the Brain Systems of Lust, Romantic Attraction, and Attachment." Archives of Sexual Behavior*, 31(5), 413-19.
50. Fisher, H. (2000). Lust, attraction, attachment: Biology and evolution of the three primary emotion systems for mating, reproduction, and parenting. *Journal of Sex Education and Therapy*, 25(1), 96-104.
51. Beck, J. G., McNiff, J., Clapp, J. D., Olsen, S. A., Avery, M. L., & Hagewood, J. H. (2011). Exploring negative emotion in women experiencing intimate partner violence: Shame, guilt, and PTSD. *Behavior therapy*, 42(4), 740-750.

52. Fabricius, W. V., & Luecken, L. J. (2007). Postdivorce living arrangements, parent conflict, and long-term physical health correlates for children of divorce. *Journal of family psychology*, 21(2), 195.

LATE ADOLESCENCE AND YOUNG ADULTS

1. Arbyn, M., & Xu, L. (2018). Efficacy and safety of prophylactic HPV vaccines. A Cochrane review of randomized trials. *Expert Review of Vaccines*, 17(12), 1085-1091.
2. Lipovac, K., Đerić, M., Tešić, M., Andrić, Z., & Marić, B. (2017). Mobile phone use while driving-literary review. *Transportation research part F: traffic psychology and behaviour*, 47, 132-142.
3. Connolly, M. D., Zervos, M. J., Barone II, C. J., Johnson, C. C., & Joseph, C. L. (2016). The mental health of transgender youth: Advances in understanding. *Journal of Adolescent Health*, 59(5), 489-495.
4. Hilton Jr, D. L. (2013). Pornography addiction–a supranormal stimulus considered in the context of neuroplasticity. *Socioaffective Neuroscience & Psychology*, 3(1), 20767.
5. Taylor, S., McKay, D., & Abramowitz, J. S. (2012). Hypochondriasis and Health-Related Anxiety. *Handbook of Evidence-Based Practice in Clinical Psychology*, 2.
6. Olatunji, B. O., Davis, M. L., Powers, M. B., & Smits, J. A. (2013). Cognitive-behavioral therapy for obsessive-compulsive disorder: A meta-analysis of treatment outcome and moderators. *Journal of psychiatric research*, 47(1), 33-41.
7. Foa, E. B., & McLean, C. P. (2016). The efficacy of exposure therapy for anxiety-related disorders and its underlying mechanisms: The case of OCD and PTSD. *Annual Review of Clinical Psychology*, 12, 1-28.
8. Nomaguchi, K. M., & Brown, S. L. (2011). Parental Strains and Rewards among Mothers: The Role of Education. *Journal of marriage and the family*, 73(3), 621–636. https://doi.org/10.1111/j.1741-3737.2011.00835.x
9. Parkes A, Sweeting H, Wight D. Parenting stress and parent support among mothers with high and low education. J Fam Psychol. 2015 Dec;29(6):907-18. doi: 10.1037/fam0000129. Epub 2015 Jul 20. PMID: 26192130; PMCID: PMC4671474.
10. De Bellis, M. D., Narasimhan, A., Thatcher, D. L., Keshavan, M. S., Soloff, P., & Clark, D. B. (2005). Prefrontal cortex, thalamus, and cerebellar volumes in adolescents and young adults with adolescent-onset alcohol use disorders and comorbid mental disorders. *Alcoholism: Clinical and Experimental Research*, 29(9), 1590-1600.
11. De Bellis, M. D., Clark, D. B., Beers, S. R., Soloff, P. H., Boring, A. M., Hall, J., ... &Keshavan, M. S. (2000). Hippocampal volume in adolescent-onset alcohol use disorders. *American Journal of Psychiatry*, 157(5), 737-744.
12. Chassin, L., Pitts, S. C., & Prost, J. (2002). Binge drinking trajectories from adolescence to emerging adulthood in a high-risk sample: predictors and substance abuse outcomes. *Journal of consulting and clinical psychology*, 70(1), 67.
13. Mehler, P. S. (2011). Medical complications of bulimia nervosa and their treatments. *International Journal of Eating Disorders*, 44(2), 95-104.

14. Casiero, D., &Frishman, W. H. (2006). Cardiovascular complications of eating disorders. *Cardiology in review*, 14(5), 227-231.
15. Fiorentini, A., Sara Volonteri, L., Dragogna, F., Rovera, C., Maffini, M., Carlo Mauri, M., & A Altamura, C. (2011). Substance-induced psychoses: a critical review of the literature. *Current drug abuse reviews*, 4(4), 228-240.
16. Radhakrishnan, R., Wilkinson, S. T., & D'Souza, D. C. (2014). Gone to pot–a review of the association between cannabis and psychosis. *Frontiers in psychiatry*, 5, 54.
17. Schimmelmann, B. G., Walger, P., & Schultze-Lutter, F. (2013). The significance of at-risk symptoms for psychosis in children and adolescents. *The Canadian Journal of Psychiatry*, 58(1), 32-40.
18. Arseneault, L., Cannon, M., Fisher, H. L., Polanczyk, G., Moffitt, T. E., & Caspi, A. (2011). Childhood trauma and children's emerging psychotic symptoms: a genetically sensitive longitudinal cohort study. *American Journal of Psychiatry*, 168(1), 65-72.
19. Duffy, M. E., Gai, A. R., Rogers, M. L., Joiner, T. E., Luby, J. L., Joshi, P. T., ... & Axelson, D. (2019). Psychotic symptoms and suicidal ideation in child and adolescent bipolar I disorder. *Bipolar disorders*, 21(4), 342-349.
20. Lundh, L. G., Wångby-Lundh, M., Paaske, M., Ingesson, S., & Bjärehed, J. (2011). Depressive symptoms and deliberate self-harm in a community sample of adolescents: a prospective study. *Depression research and treatment*, 2011.
21. Peh, C. X., Shahwan, S., Fauziana, R., Mahesh, M. V., Sambasivam, R., Zhang, Y., ... & Subramaniam, M. (2017). Emotion dysregulation as a mechanism linking child maltreatment exposure and self-harm behaviors in adolescents. *Child abuse & neglect*, 67, 383-390.
22. Barrett, K. C., Ashley, R., Strait, D. L., & Kraus, N. (2013). Art and science: how musical training shapes the brain. *Frontiers in Psychology*, 4, 713.
23. Campbell, J. C., Webster, D., Koziol-McLain, J., Block, C., Campbell, D., Curry, M. A., Gary, F., Glass, N., McFarlane, J., Sachs, C., Sharps, P., Ulrich, Y., Wilt, S. A., Manganello, J., Xu, X., Schollenberger, J., Frye, V., & Laughon, K. (2003). Risk factors for femicide in abusive relationships: results from a multisite case control study. *American journal of public health*, 93(7), 1089–1097. https://doi.org/10.2105/ajph.93.7.1089
24. Kellermann, A. L., & Mercy, J. A. (1992). Men, women, and murder: gender-specific differences in rates of fatal violence and victimization. *The Journal of Trauma*, 33(1), 1-5.
25. Sorenson, S. B. (2006). Firearm use in intimate partner violence: A brief overview. *Evaluation Review*, 30(3), 229-236.
26. Waaktaar, T., Kan, K. J., & Torgersen, S. (2018). The genetic and environmental architecture of substance use development from early adolescence into young adulthood: A longitudinal twin study of comorbidity of alcohol, tobacco and illicit drug use. *Addiction*, 113(4), 740-748.

Made in the USA
Columbia, SC
07 October 2021

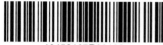